M000284141

*The*
# GUIDEBOOK

# *of* Sexual
# Medicine

# *The* GUIDEBOOK

# *of* Sexual Medicine

## WAGUIH WILLIAM ISHAK, MD, FAPA

*Editor and Author*

Director, Psychiatry Residency Training Program
Medical Director, Adult Outpatient Psychiatry Service
Cedars-Sinai Medical Center
Clinical Assistant Professor of Psychiatry
University of California at Los Angeles
David Geffen School of Medicine
Los Angeles, California

The Guidebook of Sexual Medicine

A&W Publishing Group
Beverly Hills, California

AWPublishing@mac.com

Copyright © 2008 Waguih William IsHak, MD, FAPA

All rights reserved. No part of this book may be reproduced by any mechanical, photographic, or electronic process, or in the form of a phonographic recording, nor may it be stored in a retrieval system, transmitted, or otherwise be copied for public or private use without prior written permission from the publisher.

Medicine is an ever-changing field. The information contained in this guidebook is subject to change without notice. Best efforts have been utilized to accomplish accuracy of information. However, the information within cannot be guaranteed for completeness and full accuracy. Prescribers need always to verify indications, dosing and side effect profiles with independent sources. In no event shall the publisher, editor, or authors be liable for any damage arising from the use of this guidebook.

ISBN: 978-0-9797410-0-5

Cover and Interior Design: Desktop Miracles, Inc.

Printed in the United States of America

Publisher's Cataloging-In-Publication Data
(Prepared by The Donohue Group, Inc.)


IsHak, Waguih William, 1964-
    The guidebook of sexual medicine / Waguih William IsHak.
        p. : ill. ;   cm.
    Includes bibliographical references and index.
    ISBN: 978-0-9797410-0-5
    1. Sexual disorders—Treatment—Handbooks, manuals, etc.   2. Sex (Psychology)—Handbooks, manuals, etc.   I. Title.   II. Title: Sexual medicine
RC556 .I84   2007

                                                        616.85/83

*To the love of my life, the amazing*
Asbasia (Hanan) Mikhail-IsHak, M.D., FACEP
*and the fruits of our love* William *and* Michael

*To the marvelous father:*
William Makram IsHak, M.D.
*may he rest in peace*

*To the magnificent mother:*
Nawara Yacoub Dawoud-IsHak, M.D.

*To the extraordinary brother:*
Rafik William IsHak, M.D., FRCS

*To the loving parents-in-law:*
Mr. and Mrs. Aboelkhair and Aziza Mikhail

*To the caring brother/sister in-law:*
Dr. and Mrs. Albert and Amanda Mikhail

*For their inspiration, encouragement, and love.*

# Acknowledgments

I gratefully acknowledge the professional contributions, guidance, and invaluable advice given by **Robert Pechnick, Ph.D.,** the champion of understanding basic science mechanisms as they relate to the clinical world, and a key supporter in the creation and finalization of this book, **Louis Ignarro, Ph.D., the Nobel Prize Winner** for breakthrough discoveries in this field, **Bertina Baer, LCSW, Ph.D.,** my first clinical supervisor, **Laura Berman, LCSW, Ph.D.,** my first co-therapist in sex therapy, **Uri Peles, M.D.** with his exceptional teaching in this area. I would like to thank **Daniel Berman, M.D.** for his unrelenting faithful trust in science and young scientists, **Irwin Goldstein, M.D.,** for his encouragement of creative interventions, and **Mark Rapaport, M.D.,** for his strong support of publishing this volume.

I am eternally indebted to **Norman Sussman, M.D.,** for giving me the opportunity of a lifetime to train at NYU. I continue to value on daily basis the priceless mentorship of **Virginia Sadock, M.D.,** who taught me most of what I know about this field, **Benjamin Sadock, M.D.,** who showed me not only how to scientifically write and edit but also how to create, **Carol Bernstein, M.D.,** who demonstrated to me how to move mountains (and move them swiftly!), **Manuel Trujillo, M.D.,** who taught me how to stand for, defend, and materialize world-changing ideas, **Brian Ladds, M.D.,** who shared with me, competently and generously, his savoir-faire (know how) about science, management, and life issues, and **Lloyd Sederer, M.D.,** who provided me graciously with invaluable guidance about book making in addition to precious career advice.

Exceptional scientists and clinicians assisted in the critique, support, and amelioration of particular chapters. I would like to thank **Shlomo Melmed, M.D.,** for his brilliant revision of the chapter on Orgasmic Disorders, **Glenn Braunstein, M.D.,** for his superb work on the chapter on Sexual Desire Disorders, and **Aelred Boyle, M.D.,** for her great suggestions regarding the introduction, and other parts of the book.

I was inspired, given growth opportunities and learned a great deal from teachers, clinicians, and leaders over the years and I gratefully acknowledge my debt to them, as they have contributed in a fundamental way (albeit indirectly) to the creation of this volume. I would like to express my gratitude to (chronologically):

William Makram IsHak, M.D.
Sir Magdi Yacoub, M.D., FRCS
Monsieur Nagy Habib
Mr. Shafik Yacoub Dawoud
Mr. Nabil Morcos
Mr. George IsHak
Mr. Ibrahim El-Betout
Professor Ahmad Abouelmagd
Prof. Dr. Adel Fawzy
Dean Hashem Fouad
Director Youssef Chahine
Professor Dr. Yehia El-Rakhawy
Dr. Salah Shaheen
Dr. Abdeen
Dr. Emad Hamdy Ghoz
Dr. Tarek Gawad
Dr. Abdelhameed Hashem
Dr. Nahed Khairy
Dr. Zeinab Nasser
Dr. Zakaria Halim
Dr. Samir Abouelmagd
Dr. Soad Moussa
Dr. Mohamed Salah
Professor Dr. Refaat Mahfouz
Professor Dr. Hassib El-Defrawi
Dr. Ahmad Abdallah
Dr. Yehia Gaafar
Mr. Kamel Morcos
Dr. Salwa Girgis
Khaled Mohamed, M.D.
Mary-Terez and Samy Rizk, M.D.
George Simpson, M.D.
Robert Cancro, M.D.
Robert Delgado, M.D.
David Nardacci, M.D.
Zebulon Taintor, M.D.
Martin Kahn, M.D.

Richard Hanson, M.D.
Burt Angrist, M.D.
Eric Peselow, M.D.
Samuel Slipp, M.D.
Maged Habib, M.D.
Greg Alsip, M.D.
Bruce Rubenstein, M.D.
Cliff Feldman, M.D., J.D.
Gary Gosselin, M.D.
Phill Halamandaris, M.D.
Laura M. O'Brien, CSW
Mr. Kim Hopper
Eugene West, M.D.
Linda Carter, Ph.D.
Martha Scotzin, Ph.D.
Morton Rubinstein, M.D.
Leonard Adler, M.D.
Marc Waldman, M.D.
Howard Silbert, M.D.
Richard Oberfield, M.D.
Asher Aladjem, M.D.
Victor Schwatrz, M.D.
Myrl Manley, M.D.
Henry Weinstein , M.D.
Howard Welsh, M.D.
Murray Alpert, Ph.D.
George Nicklin, M.D.
Arthur Meyerson, M.D.
Mr. Ben Goldhagen
Mr. J.J. Larrea
Jean Endicott, Ph.D.
Mr. Frank Schorn
Peter Goertz, M.D.
Bruce Levine, M.D.
Tal Burt, M.D.
Michael Welner, M.D.
Henry Chung, M.D.

Laura Roberts, M.D.
Danni Michaeli, M.D.
Victor Rodack, M.D.
Julie Pierce, M.D.
Michelle Montemayor, M.D.
Michael Sobel, M.D.
Ayman Fanous, M.D.
Abdullah Hassan, M.D.
Manuel Santos, M.D.
Patrick Callahan, Ph.D.
Russell Lim, M.D.
A. John Rush, M.D.
Sherwyn Woods, M.D.
Peter Panzarino, M.D.
Jeffrey Wilkins, M.D.
Syed Naqvi, M.D.
Russell Poland, Ph.D.

Thomas Trott, M.D., Ph.D.
Saul Brown, M.D.
Frank Williams, M.D.
Lev Gertsik, M.D.
Father Michael Gabriel
Ms. Yvonne Neely
Andrea Rogers, LCSW
Richard Rosenthal, M.D.
Thomas Rosko, M.D.
Daniel Winstead, M.D.
Ira Lesser, M.D.
Robert Cohen, M.D., Ph.D.
Ernst Schwarz, M.D., Ph.D.
Nima Fahimian, M.D.
Anne Peters, M.D.
Margi Stuber, M.D.
Fawzy I. Fawzy, M.D.

**I was supported, guided, and encouraged over the years by (chronologically)**

**In Port Said, Egypt**

Dr. Montasser El-Ghoz
Dr. Mohsen El-Ghoz
Mr. Samy Abdelazim

Mr. Mohamed El-Masry
Mr. Abdou Raafat Awad
Mr. Ayman Rashad

**At Cairo University School of Medicine**

Reda Girgis, M.D.
Ayman Tadros, M.D.
Dr. Shamel Hashem
Dr. Nabil Raguai
Dr. Tamer Goueli
Dr. Mohamed Foda
Dr. Cherif Abdel-Al
Dr. Nehad El-Mekawy
Dr. Wael Gawad
Dr. Amr Wael Farag

Dr. George Milad
Nancy Hanna, M.D.
Dr. Hussein Gohar
Dr. Hossam El-Gamal
Dr. Adel Badr
Dr. Bassel Ebeid
Dr. Hala Fakhry
Dr. Amr El-Shabrawishy
Dr. Ashraf Ramadan
Dr. Wael Sakr

**At Dar El-Mokattum Milieu Therapy Hospital, Cairo**

Drs. Aref and Manal Khweiled
Mr. Mustafa Hassan
Dr. Sayed and Ms. Olfat El-Refayi
Dr. Ahmad Hussein
Ms. Mai El-Rakhawy
Ms. Iman Abdelatif
Ms. Marlene Sedky

Dr. Nabil El-Kot
Dr. Monsef Mahfouz
Mr. Mohamed Salama
Dr. Nagy Gamil
Dr. Liliane Helmy
Dr. Ibrahim

At NYU Psychiatry Residency Program

| | |
|---|---|
| Doug Fogelman, M.D. | Fidel Ventura, M.D. |
| Jose DeAsis, M.D. | Paulina Loo, M.D. |
| Holly Schwartz, M.D. | Antonio Abad, M.D. |
| Samoon Ahmad, M.D. | Elyse Weiner, M.D. |
| Marylinn Markarian, M.D. | Adarsh Gupta, M.D. |
| Peter Sass, M.D. | Ann Maloney, M.D. |
| Stacey Lane, M.D. | John Heussy, M.D. |

**I wanted to thank my authors and co-authors for their valuable contributions especially (alphabetically if not mentioned above)**

| | |
|---|---|
| Rod Amiri, M.D. | Lucy Postolov, L.Ac., Dipl. Ac. |
| Natalya Bussel, M.D. | Hesham Shafik, M.D. |
| Manar ElBohy, M.D. | Stephanie Michael Stewart, M.D. |
| Elizabeth (Dee) Hartmann, P.T. | Monisha Vasa, M.D. |
| William Huang, M.D. | Elizabeth L. Wood, LSW |
| Kerrie Grow McLean, Psy.D. | Jay Yew, M.D. |
| Albert Mikhail, M.D. | |

We (editor and authors) are also indebted to the **American Psychiatric Association** for permission to reproduce copyright material related to diagnostic criteria of sexual disorders, and **Dr. Z.H. Cho** for the exceptional graphs about acupuncture. Several people have been instrumental in allowing this project to be completed. I would like to especially thank **Penny Callmeyer, Barry Kerrigan, Del LeMond, Susan Clark,** and the staff at **Desktop Miracles** for their outstanding professional work and patience throughout the duration of this project.

This book is dedicated to the medical students, residents, and faculty at the **Departments of Psychiatry at Cairo University School of Medicine, Dar El-Mokattum Milieu Therapy Hospital, New York University School of Medicine (NYU), University of California at Los Angeles School of Medicine (UCLA), and Cedars-Sinai Medical Center.**

WAGUIH WILLIAM ISHAK, MD, FAPA

# Table of Contents

FOREWORD     xv

*Louis Ignarro, Ph.D., Nobel Prize Winner in Medicine*

## Introduction and History of Sexual Medicine     1

*Waguih William IsHak, M.D.*

## CHAPTER 1 The Sexual Response Cycle     7

*Waguih William IsHak, M.D., and Monisha Vasa, M.D.*

## CHAPTER 2 Biopsychosocial Evaluation and Treatment of Sexual Disorders     21

*Waguih William IsHak, M.D.*

## CHAPTER 3 Substance-Induced Sexual Disorders     43

*Waguih William IsHak, M.D., Stephanie Stewart, M.D., Robert Pechnick, Ph.D., William Huang, M.D., and Ernst Schwarz, M.D., Ph.D.*

## CHAPTER 4 Sexual Disorders Due to General Medical Conditions     67

*Waguih William IsHak, M.D., Shahrad Rod Amiri, M.D., and Ernst Schwarz, M.D., Ph.D.*

## CHAPTER 5 Sexual Desire Disorders     87

*Waguih William IsHak, M.D., and Aelred Boyle, M.D.*

## CHAPTER 6 Sexual Arousal Disorders     103

*Albert Mikhail, M.D., and Jay Yew, M.D.*

CHAPTER 7 **Orgasmic Disorders** 125
*Waguih William IsHak, M.D., Laura Berman, Ph.D.,*
*and Kerrie Grow McLean, Psy.D.*

CHAPTER 8 **Sexual Pain Disorders** 149
*Manar ElBohy, M.D., Hesham Shafik, M.D.,*
*and Waguih William IsHak, M.D.*

CHAPTER 9 **Alternative Medicine in Sexual**
**Performance Enhancement** 173
*Lucy Postolov, L.Ac.*

CHAPTER 10 **Women's Sexual Health** 191
*Laura Berman, LCSW, Ph.D., Dee Hartmann, PT,*
*Elizabeth L. Wood, LSW,*

APPENDIX I **Summary of Sex Surveys Findings** 215
*Natalya Bussel, M.D.*

APPENDIX II **Online Screening Tests for Sexual Disorders** 225
*Waguih William IsHak, M.D.*

APPENDIX III **The DSM-IV in a Nutshell:** 229
**A Practical Approach to Psychiatric Diagnosis**
*Waguih William IsHak, M.D., Eugene Lee, M.D.,*
*Ravi Bhalavat, M.D., Monisha Vasa, M.D.*

# List of Contributors

**Rod Amiri, M.D.**
Psychiatry Residency Training Program
Cedars-Sinai Medical Center
Los Angeles, California

**Laura Berman, Ph.D.**
Assistant Clinical Professor of Obstetrics,
    Gynecology and Psychiatry
Feinberg School of Medicine,
    Northwestern University
Director, Berman Center
Chicago, Illinois

**Ravi Bhalavat, M.D.**
Department of Psychiatry
Cedars-Sinai Medical Center
Los Angeles, California

**Aelred Boyle, M.D.**
Assistant Professor of Psychiatry
Albert Einstein College of Medicine
Medical Director, Bronx Lebanon
    Hospital
Bronx, New York

**Natalya Bussel, M.D.**
Department of Psychiatry
University of California at Los Angeles
David Geffen School of Medicine
Los Angeles, California

**Manar ElBohy, M.D.**
Attending Psychiatrist
Psychological Medicine Hospital
Kuwait City, Kuwait

**Elizabeth (Dee) Hartmann, P.T.**
    **(Physical Therapist)**
Berman Center
Chicago, Illinois

**William Huang, M.D.**
Department of Psychiatry
Cedars-Sinai Medical Center
Los Angeles, California

**Louis Ignarro, Ph.D.**
Nobel Laureate
Professor of Pharmacology
University of California at Los Angeles
David Geffen School of Medicine at
    UCLA
Los Angeles, California

**Waguih William IsHak, M.D.**
Director, Psychiatry Residency Training
    Program
Medical Director, Adult Outpatient
    Psychiatry Service
Cedars-Sinai Medical Center
Assistant Clinical Professor of Psychiatry
University of California at Los Angeles
David Geffen School of Medicine at
    UCLA
Los Angeles, California

**Kerrie Grow McLean, Psy.D.**
Psychologist, Independent Practice
Chicago, Illinois

**Eugene Lee, M.D.**
Psychiatry Residency Program
Cedars-Sinai Medical Center
Los Angeles, California

**Albert Mikhail, M.D.**
Department of Urology
Kaiser Permanente
Fontana, California

**Robert Pechnick, Ph.D.**
Professor of Psychiatry
University of California at Los Angeles
David Geffen School of Medicine
Associate Director, Psychiatric Research
Cedars-Sinai Medical Center
Los Angeles, California

**Lucy Postolov, L.Ac., Dipl. Ac.**
   **(Acupuncturist)**
Director, Postolova Acupuncture Group
Director, Integrated Medicine program,
   Glendale Memorial Hospital
Allied Health Professional, Cedars-Sinai
   Medical Center
Los Angeles, California

**Hesham Shafik, M.D.**
Attending Psychiatrist
Psychological Medicine Hospital
Kuwait City, Kuwait

**Ernst Schwarz, M.D., Ph.D.**
Division of Cardiology
Cedars-Sinai Medical Center
Professor of Medicine
University of California at Los Angeles
David Geffen School of Medicine
Los Angeles, California

**Stephanie Michael Stewart, M.D.**
Psychiatry Residency Training Program
Cedars-Sinai Medical Center
Los Angeles, California

**Monisha Vasa, M.D.**
Psychiatry Residency Training Program
Cedars-Sinai Medical Center
Los Angeles, California

**Elizabeth L. Wood, LSW**
Berman Center
Chicago, Illinois

**Jay Yew, M.D.**
Department of Urology
Sharp Memorial Hospital
San Diego, California

# Foreword

LOUIS IGNARRO

Medical discoveries are often the result of long, repeated, and persistent attempts at testing hypotheses in an environment where biomedical research is at times impeded by methodological, financial, and administrative limitations and pressures. However, the creative task of piecing together findings that appear unconnected to each other, and at times are generated from various fields, pose the most significant challenge. Breakthrough discoveries are often a mix of scientific rigor, collaboration, and serendipity. The discovery of the role of nitric oxide (NO) as a key signaling molecule in biology is no different.

Practical and originally unforeseen applications of this discovery are still evolving and have unlimited potential in the treatment of cardiovascular and other diseases. The discovery of NO led to the elucidation of the fundamental mechanisms underlying penile erection. Moreover, it heralded the development and introduction of the first orally active agent to effectively treat erectile disorders. This breakthrough has enhanced the lives and relationships of millions of people globally. If sex is the ultimate physical expression of love, one could see that persistent problems in sexual performance impair one of the fundamental roles in the human experience. Restoration of sexual health hence becomes an essential factor not only in health promotion but also in quality of life improvement.

*The Guidebook of Sexual Medicine* is a practical manual for clinicians of all sorts of professional backgrounds who are charged with evaluation and treatment of sexual disorders. This volume underscores the value of an in-depth exploration of biological and psychosocial factors underlying sexual dysfunction, and widens the scope of interventions by highlighting the importance of integrating biological and psychosocial treatments. It also calls attention to "the couple" as a core unit in restoration of sexual health and quality of life enhancement.

As more discoveries are underway, I am certain that scientific breakthroughs will continue to offer more solutions to complicated health problems, bringing to an end the suffering of many people worldwide.

LOUIS IGNARRO, PH.D.
NOBEL LAUREATE

# Introduction and History of Sexual Medicine

WAGUIH WILLIAM ISHAK, M.D.

## I. Introduction

Kolodny, Masters and Johnson coined the term sexual medicine in their well-known *Textbook of Sexual Medicine* (Kolodny, Masters and Johnson 1979). Sexual medicine is the branch of medicine that focuses on the evaluation and treatment of sexual disorders, which have a high prevalence rate, affecting about 43% of women and 31% of men (Rosen 2000).

The brain is involved in controlling complex cognitive, affective, and physiological factors influencing sexual function (Bancroft 1988). The biochemical mechanisms involving desire and arousal are only partially understood, but it is assumed that they have two components: a set of central mechanisms; and another set of peripheral ones. The central supraspinal systems are mainly localized in the limbic system (olfactory nuclei, nucleus accumbens, amygdala, hippocampus, etc.) and in the hypothalamus and its nuclei (paraventricular preoptic, and ventromedial nuclei). Neural information travels through the brain stem, the medulla oblongata, the spinal cord and the autonomous nervous system to the genital apparatus. Very little is known of the central mechanisms involved. Nevertheless, several neurotransmitters and neuropeptides, such as dopamine, glutamic acid, nitric oxide, oxytocin, ACTH-MSH peptides, are known to facilitate

1

sexual function, while serotonin, gamma-aminobutyric acid (GABA) and opioid peptides reduce it.

In March 1998 the phosphodiesterase-5 (PDE-5) inhibitor sildenafil (Viagra) became the first oral drug approved by the FDA for the treatment of male erectile disorder and the drug is reported to have helped more than 16 million men.

Sales of sildenafil reach 1.5 billion dollars annually and 9 pills are dispensed every second! This groundbreaking discovery largely credited to the pioneering work of Louis Ignarro was recognized with a Nobel Prize award. It has opened the door for the development of newer drugs in this class, such as vardenafil (Levitra) and tadalafil (Cialis). Newer pharmacological agents are currently under investigation (Goldhill 2002).

Perhaps because of these immense strides in pharmacology, psychological treatments, including couples counseling, have been falling out of vogue and are becoming (in the psychiatric community, at least) a last resort when drugs are ineffective. Fewer and fewer practitioners are addressing these sensitive issues in the context of the couple. It is not totally clear how clinicians have gradually neglected that "it takes two!" and that sex education and communication between the two partners are more vital to a healthy sex life than just an erect penis achieved by the use of PDE-5 inhibitors.

This volume integrates biological and psychological schools of thought by using a biopsychosocial approach to the evaluation and treatment of sexual dysfunction, with significant emphasis on the couple. The Biopsychosocial model ensures a comprehensive assessment of multiple factors (psychosocial, medical, and the effect of substances) that can affect sexual functioning, so that the individual and/or the couple can benefit from different types of interventions, whether they are biological, psychosocial, or both (IsHak et al. 2005). The current model of the sexual response cycle is discussed in chapter 1. A discussion of the Biopsychosocial evaluation and Biopsychosocial treatments of sexual disorders is covered in chapter 2. The following two chapters (3 and 4) describe substance-induced sexual dysfunction and sexual disorders caused by medical conditions. Chapters 5 through 8 deal with disorders of desire, arousal, orgasm, and pain. Chapter 9 focuses on alternative medicine interventions in sexual performance enhancement, while chapter 10 is dedicated to women's sexual health. This volume ends with an appendix on the results of sex surveys and another on the available online screening tests for sexual disorders in women and men. Paraphilias and gender identity disorders are related topics that are beyond the scope of this manual and are not covered here.

## II. History of Sexual Medicine

One of the first sex manuals in history is the Kama Sutra, written in India, in second century B.C. Techniques of sexual pleasure enhancement including positions are fully explained including the spiritual aspects.

In 1896, Havelock Ellis, an English physician, published "Studies in the Psychology of Sex", discussing normal and abnormal sexuality. Around the same time, in 1898, Richard von Krafft-Ebing, a German psychiatrist, published in Latin a book called *Psychopathia Sexualis* which is the first modern text on sexual disorders including the Paraphilias.

By 1918, Sigmund Freud, the founder of psychoanalysis, considered sexuality central to his psychoanalytic theory. Early in the 20th century, German physician Magnus Hirshfeld founded the first sex-research institute in Germany. He conducted the first large-scale sex survey, collecting data from 10,000 men and women. He also initiated the first journal for publishing the results of sex studies. The Nazis destroyed most of his materials during World War. In the early 1930's American anthropologist Margaret Mead and British anthropologist Bronislav Malinowsky began studying sexual behavior in different cultures (Sanders 2006).

In the United States Alfred Kinsey, published a survey of 18,000 subjects regarding sexual behaviors in 1947. William Masters and Virginia Johnson followed this survey with rigorous lab study of sexual encounters. Masters and Johnson developed key concepts in sexual medicine such the sexual response cycle, and developed an effective treatment techniques for sexual dysfunction such as sex therapy.

The National Health and Social Life Survey (NHSLS), the Chicago Study or Chicago Survey, was published in Sex in America: a Definitive Survey (Michael et al. 1994), and The Social Organization of Sexuality (Laumann et al. 1994). Randomly selected 3,432 subjects underwent a face-to-face survey. This well-designed survey revealed that about 43% of women and 31% of men are suffering from sexual dysfunction. The specific findings of the prevalence of each specific disorder are listed in the Epidemiology section in each. More findings from this survey are highlighted in Appendix I.

The most significant breakthrough was the identification of nitric oxide as the principle neurotransmitter responsible for the relaxation of the corpus cavernosum smooth muscle, by Louis Ignarro, Ph.D. in 1997, as a result of two decades of research (Ignarro 1998). This discovery enabled the development of oral pharmacological agents for the treatment of erectile dysfunction. Dr. Ignarro was awarded the Nobel Prize for this momentous discovery in 1998.

The late 1990s brought more focus on women's sexual health, largely due to the efforts of Jennifer and Laura Berman who were originally mentored by Irwin Goldstein at Boston University (Berman et al. 2001).

The current state of the field is an exciting one, with a plethora of biochemical and physical interventions, in addition to well-tested and effective psychosocial ones. The next focus is going to be 'the couple' as the main hub of the efforts to improve sexual functioning and subsequently quality of life.

# *References*

Bancroft J: Sexual desire and the brain. Sexual & Marital Therapy Vol 3(1) 11-27, 1988

Berman J, Berman L, Bumiller E: For Women Only: A Revolutionary Guide to Overcoming Sexual Dysfunction and Reclaiming Your Sex Life. Henry Holt Company, New York NY, 2001

Goldhill J: Male and female sexual dysfunction: Blockbuster indication for multiple pharmacological targets. LeadDiscovery Ltd, http://www.leaddiscovery.co.uk/target-discovery/abstracts/dossier-MDI002.html, 2002

Ignarro L: Nitric Oxide: A Unique Endogenous Signaling Molecule in Vascular Biology. Nobel Lecture, December 8, 1998, posted in full text at http://nobelprize.org/nobel_prizes/medicine/laureates/1998/ignarro-lecture.pdf, 1998

IsHak WW, Mikhail AA, Amiri SR, Berman L, and Vasa M: Sexual Dysfunction. Focus 3:520-525, 2005

Kolodny RC, Masters WH, and Johnson VE: Textbook of sexual medicine. Boston, MA, Little Brown, 1979

Laumann EO, Gagnon JH, Michael RT, and Michaels S: The Social Organization of Sexuality: Sexual Practices in the United States. Chicago, IL, University of Chicago Press, 1994

Masters and Johnson, Human Sexual Response. Boston, Little Brown, 1966

Masters WH: Homosexuality in Perspective. Baltimore, MD, Lippincott Williams & Wilkins, 1979

Masters WH: Human Sexual Inadequacy. Baltimore, MD, Lippincott Williams & Wilkins, 1970

Michael RT, Gagnon JH, Laumann EO, and Kolata G: Sex in America: a Definitive Survey. New York, NY, Little Brown, 1994

Rosen RC: Prevalence and risk factors of sexual dysfunction in men and women. Current Psychiatry Reports 2(3):189-95, 2000

Sanders SA: Human Sexuality in Microsoft Encarta Online Encyclopedia, http://encarta.msn.com, 2006

# 1

# Sexual Response Cycle

WAGUIH WILLIAM ISHAK, M.D.
MONISHA VASA, M.D.

## I. Introduction

The sexual response cycle gives us a framework for examining the physical changes that men and women experience in a sexual interaction. It is critical to understand the current definition of the sexual response cycle, as well as historically how the current model developed. We can use our understanding of "normal" sexual function to then define sexual "dysfunction" and disorders.

Sigmund Freud was one of the earliest thinkers who considered sexual response as a sequence of related events (Leiblum 2000). Freud wrote "the execution of the sex act presupposes a very complicated sequence of events, any one of which may be the locus of disturbance" (Freud 1936). The details of that sequence of events were first fleshed out by the pioneering studies of Masters and Johnson, who studied the micro details of 14,000 sexual encounters over two decades. The data was published in their famous text, "Human Sexual Response" in 1966.

Masters and Johnson described the sexual response cycle as a linear sequence of four stages that both men and women experienced, despite different anatomy and physiology (Masters and Johnson 1966):

1. Excitement
2. Plateau
3. Orgasm
4. Resolution

This model became the basis for the diagnosis and classification of sexual disorders in both the 1980 and 1987 DSM-III and DSM III-R respectively. However, as clinicians became adept at using the response cycle to understand dysfunction, it became evident that there was a key missing piece. A great deal of patients presented with problems of low interest, desire, or libido, a stage that had not been adequately described in the Masters and Johnson model. Furthermore, although the stages of plateau and resolution were descriptive, there were not many disorders associated with these two phases (Leiblum 2000).

A decade later, Helen Singer Kaplan, a psychiatrist and professor of sex therapy, developed a triphasic model that addressed these concerns. She added the initiating phase of desire, and eliminated the phases of plateau and resolution:

1. Desire
2. Arousal
3. Orgasm

Sexual disorders are organized according to the above triphasic model in the DSM-IV-TR, leading to Sexual Desire Disorders, Sexual Arousal Disorders, and Sexual Orgasm Disorders, with the additional category of Sexual Pain Disorders (APA 2000).

Therefore, between the Masters and Johnson model and the Kaplan model, there are five stages that collectively describe the sexual response in men and women. Although Kaplan's model is the currently accepted theory, it is helpful to study the details of all five stages to gain a complete understanding of the sexual interaction.

1. Desire (also called libido): This stage is characterized by wanting or desiring sexual intimacy or gratification.

2. Arousal (also called excitement): This stage is characterized by the body's initial response to feelings of sexual desire. This manifests by erection in males and lubrication in females.

3. Plateau: This stage is the highest point of sexual excitement, where arousal is maintained at a maximal intensity leading to the next stage of orgasm.

4. Orgasm: This stage is the peak of the plateau stage where sexual tension is released, and is manifested by pleasurable rhythmic contractions of parts of the genital organs.

5. Resolution: This stage is when the body returns to its pre-excitement phase.

## II. Detailed Description of Known Phases of the Sexual Response Cycle

### A. Desire

Our minds and bodies can respond sexually to a variety of stimuli—including sight, sound, smell, touch, taste, movement, fantasy, and memory. These stimuli can create sexual desire—a strong wanting for stimulation (either by oneself or with another person) or intimacy that may cause one to seek sexual satisfaction. Societal and cultural values influence the range of stimuli that provoke desire, and ideas about the stimuli considered "sexual" or "attractive" can vary greatly between cultures and among subsets of a single culture. In addition, each individual reacts to sets of stimuli that are idiosyncratic—based on his or her own thoughts, feelings, and experiences. Thus, desire in a given individual is the culmination of biological factors (levels of hormones such as androgens and estrogens), cognitive factors such as the wish for sexual activity and the risk one is willing to sustain for it, and motivational factors, such as the desire for increased intimacy in a given relationship.

Desire may be communicated between potential sexual partners either verbally or through body language and behavior (for example, through "flirting"). This communication, which is shaped by sociocultural factors, may be subtle and easily misread. In different cultures, behaviors meant to communicate desire may vary greatly along gender lines; for example, in some cultures, women are expected not to express overt, verbal communication of their sexual desire, whereas such communication from men is expected.

In summary, desire is a prelude to sexual excitement and sexual activity. It occurs in the mind, rather than in the body, and may not progress to sexual excitement without further physical or mental stimulation.

## B. Excitement (Arousal)

The excitement phase described by Masters and Johnson is equivalent to the arousal phase described by Kaplan. Excitement can be viewed as the body's physical response to desire. A person who manifests the physical indications of desire is termed to be "aroused" or "excited." The progression from desire to excitement depends on a wide variety of factors—it may be brought on by sensory stimulation, thoughts, fantasy, or even the suggestion that desire may be reciprocated. For some, (particularly for some adolescents), the excitement stage may be achieved with very little physical or mental stimulation, whereas for others, significant intimacy, physical stimulation, or fantasy may be required. Excitement may lead to sexual activity, but this is not inevitable: for both sexes, initial physical excitement may be lost and regained many times without progression to the next stage. It generally takes longer for women to achieve full arousal than for men to do so.

Excitement can be communicated between partners verbally, through body language, through behavior, or through any of the following physiologic changes:

1. For both sexes: This phase is characterized by manifestations of "sexual tension." There is a generalized vasocongestion of the body, resulting in a sexual flush. Heart rate and blood pressure increase, breathing becomes heavier, and body muscles tense. The nipples become erect, genital and pelvic blood vessels become engorged, and involuntary and voluntary muscles contract.

2. For women: Vaginal lubrication is the key indicator of sexual excitement. This occurs as blood flow increases to the vaginal walls, resulting in a transudate within ten to thirty seconds of sexual stimulation. The vagina also lengthens and widens in preparation for sexual intercourse. Other changes include swelling of the breasts, clitoris, and labia. The uterus also becomes enlarged and rises in the pelvic vault.

3. For men: Erection of the penis is the key indicator of sexual excitement. Also, the scrotum thickens, and the testes rise closer to the body, secondary to shortening of the spermatic cord Men generally attain the stage of excitement faster than women do. Thus desire leads to excitement via central mechanisms, including the activation of thoughts, dreams and fantasies. Men and women manifest excitement both through non-genital peripheral mechanisms such as salivation, sweating, cutaneous vasodilatation and nipple erection, as well as genital mechanisms such as engorgement of the penis, clitoris, labia and vagina.

## C. Plateau

If physical or mental stimulation (especially stroking and rubbing of erogenous zones or sexual intercourse) continues during full arousal, the plateau stage may be achieved. This stage, the highest moment of sexual excitement before orgasm, may be achieved, lost, and regained several times without the occurrence of orgasm. Therefore, the plateau phase can be viewed as a more advanced stage of excitement or arousal, which occurs immediately prior to orgasm (Kaplan 1974).

The plateau stage can be communicated between partners verbally, through body language, through behavior, or through any of the following physiological changes:

1. For both sexes: Breathing rate, heart rate, and blood pressure further increase, sexual flush deepens, and muscle tension increases. The local vasocongestion of the genitals is at its peak in both genders. There is a sense of impending orgasm.

2. For women: The clitoris withdraws, the Bartholin's glands lubricate, the areolae around the nipples become larger, the labia continue to

swell, and the uterus tips to stand high in the abdomen. The "orgasmic platform" develops; that is, the lower vagina swells, narrows, and tightens.

3. For men: The Cowper's glands secrete pre-ejaculatory fluid. The testes engorge with blood, causing a fifty percent increase in size, and also rise closer to the body. The penis is distended with blood to its full capacity, and the ridge of the glans penis becomes more prominent.

## D. Orgasm

Orgasm occurs at the peak of the plateau phase. At the moment of orgasm, the sexual tension that has been building throughout the body is released, and the body is flooded with chemicals called endorphins, which cause a sense of well-being and intense pleasure. Orgasm can be achieved through mental stimulation and fantasy alone, but more commonly is a result of direct physical stimulation or sexual intercourse (although many women report difficulty in achieving orgasm through vaginal intercourse alone).

The intensity of orgasm can vary among individuals and can vary within an individual from one sexual experience to another. Orgasm may involve intense spasm and loss of awareness, or it may be signaled by as little as a sigh or subtle relaxation. Orgasm can be communicated between partners verbally, through body language, through behavior, or through any of the following physiological changes:

1. For both sexes: Heart rate, breathing, and blood pressure reach their highest peak, with heart rate reaching a peak of 180 beats per minute, and respiratory rate increasing to forty breaths per minute. The sexual flush spreads over the body, and there is a loss of muscle control (spasms). Myotonia may cause spasmodic contractions in the hands, feet, and face. In both genders, muscles go into spasm throughout the body with facial grimacing and clenched fists being common. Multiple sensory afferent information from trigger points such as clitoris, labia, vagina, periurethral glans, etc., are passed centrally to supraspinal structures likely involving the thalamic septum. Pleasurable sensory information is also carried to the cortical pleasure sites.

2. For women: Orgasm is usually obtained through some form of clitoral stimulation in women. During orgasm, the uterus, vagina, anus, and muscles of the pelvic floor contract five to 12 times at 0.8-second intervals and another 3–6 weaker and slower contractions may follow. The uterus and anal sphincter muscles also contract and dips the deposited sperm into the cervix.

3. For men: Ejaculation, contractions of the ejaculatory duct in the prostate gland causing semen to be ejected through the urethra and penis, occurs. The urethra, anus, and muscles of the pelvic floor contract three to six times at 0.8-second intervals after ejaculation, and are experienced as orgasm proper.

## E. Resolution

Resolution is the period following orgasm, during which muscles relax and the body begins to return to its pre-excitement state. Immediately following orgasm, men experience a refractory period, during which erection cannot be achieved. The duration of this period varies from five minutes to twenty four hours among individuals, and increases with age. Women experience no refractory period—they can either enter the resolution stage or return to the excitement or plateau stage immediately following orgasm.

Resolution can be communicated between partners verbally, through body language, through behavior, or through any of the following body changes:

1. For both sexes: Heart rate and blood pressure dip below normal, returning to normal soon afterward. In 30–40% of individuals, the whole body (including the palms of hands and soles of feet) sweats. There is a loss of muscle tension within five minutes of orgasm, followed by a generalized sense of increased relaxation and drowsiness. The sex flush lightens rapidly.

2. For women: Blood vessels dilate to drain the pelvic tissues and decrease engorgement. Subsequently, the labia return to normal color, size and position, and the clitoris shrinks slightly and resumes its pre-arousal position The cervix opens to help semen travel up into the uterus (closing 20–30 minutes after orgasm), while the

uterus lowers into the upper vagina (location of semen after male orgasm during penile-vaginal intercourse). The breasts and areolae decrease in size, and the nipples lose their erection

3. For men: The penis lightens in color and becomes softer and smaller. The scrotum relaxes, and the testes drop farther away from the body. Nipples lose their erection.

Kaplan pointed out that, although the Masters and Johnson sexual response cycle is described as a single linear sequence of events in men and women, the cycle can also be viewed as a biphasic process. In both genders, there are two distinct and independent processes occurring. The first phase is the genital vasocongestive reaction causing erection in men and vaginal lubrication in women. The second phase is the reflex clonic muscular contractions of orgasm. Kaplan felt that it was helpful to identify these different aspects of the cycle, as it clarified the underlying physiology, and the resulting pathology. For example, erection in men is mediated by the parasympathetic nervous system, while ejaculation (which occurs immediately before orgasm) is mediated by the sympathetic system. Furthermore, the vasocongestive process and the orgasmic process are affected differently by illness, drugs, and aging, and would therefore require different treatments (Kaplan 1974).

## III. The Evolution of the Sexual Response Cycle

Kaplan's triphasic model developed almost a decade after the original Masters and Johnson version secondary to deficits and criticisms about the original four-step sequence. The first criticism, as mentioned earlier, was that desire, a key factor in initiating the sexual act, was not included, while the phases of plateau and resolution, which were not associated with significant dysfunction, were included. Furthermore, during the sexual act, it was easy to identify the excitement phase in men via the presence/absence of an erection, but vaginal lubrication was not found to correlate with women's subjective sense of excitement or arousal. For example, women could have a great deal of vaginal lubrication without feeling aroused, and without being aware of the lubrication. On the other hand, many women can feel excited or aroused, without extensive lubrication. Other criticisms revolved around the idea that the Masters and Johnson cycle was phallocentric, implying that intercourse and orgasm were the only important end points of sexual interaction. Similarly, it was felt that the Masters and Johnson cycle overemphasized the physiological changes involved in the sexual act, and did not emphasize the emotional and interpersonal aspects which, to some, are key to the overall sexual experience (Leiblum 2000).

A final criticism, which persists today even with respect to the triphasic Kaplan model, is that although termed a "cycle", the sequence of events was depicted as linear, one leading to the next. Such a linear sequence more accurately describes male sexuality. However in female sexuality, the phases might occur in a different order, with each phase reinforcing and feeding back to previous phases (i.e., a more "circular model"). Many women do not spontaneously experience desire, and wait for their partners to initiate before deciding whether or not to participate. Furthermore, in many women, arousal either precedes, or cannot be separated from, desire. The triphasic Kaplan cycle of desire, arousal, and orgasm also does not include salient aspects of emotion and intimacy, or the important end point of satisfaction (Leiblum 2000).

This speaks especially to differences between female and male sexuality. Men often pursue sex for physical release of sexual urges; women, on the other hand may not always require a similar release, but often seek sex to satisfy a craving for emotional closeness and intimacy (Leiblum 2000). It is important to consider these criticisms of the sexual response cycle, as they widen our perspective and scope on sexual function and dysfunction, and broaden our understanding of what "normalcy" is in the sexual arena for men and women.

In 1999, Rosemary Basson, a psychiatrist created a new model to describe sexual response in females to address some of these gaps. Basson postulated that, based on internal or external stimuli (including nonsexual interpersonal factors), women make a conscious decision to become aroused, which then triggers sexual desire. If effective physical and emotional stimulation continues, arousal in the woman continues to build. Arousal may or may not ultimately lead to orgasm. However, if the process results in a sense of sexual satisfaction for the woman, the cycle is likely to be repeated. Thus this is a more circular description of female sexuality, removing intercourse and orgasm as a necessary end point for sexual satisfaction to be obtained (Basson 2000).

Other models to describe normal sexual function in females have also been created. Researchers such as Sugrue and Whipple discussed how female sexuality can be more complex than the presence or absence of lubrication and orgasm. Female sexual experience involves and encompasses a variety of factors, including self-esteem, body image, and relationship dynamics, akin to the "internal and external stimuli" described in the Basson model. The alternative approach that Sugrue and Whipple used involved four components:

1. **Capacity** to experience sexual pleasure and satisfaction independent of the capacity for orgasm.

2. **Desire** for, or receptivity to, sexual pleasure.

3. **Physical** capability to respond to stimulation without discomfort (vasocongestion).

4. **Capability** to experience orgasm under suitable circumstances.

If these characteristics, as part of a Biopsychosocial sexual perspective, were viewed as part of normal sexual function, the absence of one or more of these traits could be viewed as sexual dysfunction (Whipple 2001).

As clinicians, it is useful to use the current Kaplan model of desire, arousal and orgasm to understand and classify sexual disorders. More psycho-physiological studies are needed to settle the problems with the Sexual Response Cycle, especially the overlap between desire and arousal. Vroege et al. (1998) had the following suggestions for the DSM-V and ICD–11: (1) introduction of excessive (hyperactive) sexual desire in addition to diminished (hypoactive) sexual desire; (2) differentiation between genital arousal disorder and sexual excitement disorder; (3) differentiation between orgasmic disorder, anhedonic orgasm, ejaculation disorder, and premature orgasm.

Criticisms, new research, and evolving concepts and models serve to expand our understanding of sexual function and disorders. This includes understanding how men and women might be unique in terms of their sexual response. Furthermore, what is normal changes as men and women evolve through their own life cycles, affected by changes in sexual orientation, practices and preferences, medical and psychiatric illness, prescription drugs and substances, and the process of aging itself.

## IV. Sexual Response and Aging

Women and men maintain sexual desire and activity throughout their lives beyond the reproductive years. In general, the genital organs become somewhat less sensitive, and as a result, the response cycle slows down, the stages of response take longer to achieve, and the intensity of sensation may be reduced. are diminished, yet pleasurable. However, with the exception of lubrication and arousal complaints, older women actually had fewer sexual complaints than younger women. For example, younger women complained more of diminished desire and difficulty obtaining orgasm compared to older women (Clayton 2003).

Post-menopausal women experience drastic drops in estrogen and progesterone, causing physiologic changes that affect sexual function. These hormone-dependent changes include thinning of the vaginal lining, reduced elasticity, and decreased lubrication, often resulting in discomfort or pain during intercourse. Urinary incontinence may also occur because of reduced estrogen. Women may also experience a loss of libido because of reduced testosterone (EngenderHealth 2003)

Normal physiological changes include the following:

A. **Desire:** A decrease in libido may be experienced, particularly for post-menopausal women.

B. **Arousal (Excitement) and C. Plateau:**

1. In women: Women may experience delayed nipple erection, reduced labial separation and swelling, and vaginal expansion. They may demonstrate decreased elevation of the uterus. Decreased lubrication during excitement can result in increased discomfort during intercourse. Furthermore, women who have experienced multiple vaginal deliveries also exhibit amore relaxed vaginal tone, which may result in less stimulation during vaginal intercourse.

2. In men: Men may experience a longer excitement stage, and an increased interval between excitement and ejaculation, with delayed and less-firm erection. More direct stimulation may be required to achieve and maintain an erection. Men may exhibit a shorter phase of impending orgasm. They may also have delayed nipple erection, decreased pre-ejaculatory emissions, and reduced muscle tension.

D. **Orgasm:** Women experience a reduced spread of sexual flush. In men, ejaculation time is shorter, with reduced volume of ejaculate and fewer ejaculatory contractions.

E. **Resolution:** In women, there is no dilation of the cervix. Men experience a more rapid loss of erection and a significantly longer refractory period, though with a more rapid return to the pre-excitement state. Nipple erection lasts longer in both women and men after orgasm.

## V. Future Directions

From Freud to Masters and Johnson to Kaplan to Basson, the sexual response cycle continues to evolve. As we further our knowledge of what motivates men and women to have sex, as well how their minds and bodies interact and respond during the sexual act, we gain both a broader, and a deeper, understanding of sexuality and its resulting disorders. Looking ahead, there is so much more to be discovered about a fundamental human act that simultaneously perplexes and inspires us.

# *References*

Basson R: The female sexual response: a different model. J Sex Marital Ther.26:51–65, 2000

Clayton A: Sexual function and dysfunction in women. Psychiatric Clinics of North America 26:673–682, 2003

EngenderHealth: http://www.engenderhealth.com/res/onc/sexuality/response/, 2003

Freud S: The Problem of Anxiety. New York, NY: The Psychoanalytical Quarterly Press and WW Norton & Co, Inc., 1936 (Original work published 1926)

Kaplan HS: The New Sex Therapy. New York, NY: Brunner/Mazel Publications, 1974

Kaplan HS: Disorders of Sexual Desire and Other New Concepts and Techniques in Sex Therapy. New York, NY: Brunner/Mazel Publications, 1979

Leiblum SR: Redefining female sexual response. Contemporary OB/GYN, 45, 120–126, 2000

Masters W and Johnson V: Human Sexual Response Cycle. Philadelphia, PA: Lippincott Williams & Wilkins Publishers, 1966

Vroege JA, Gijs L, Hengeveld MW: Classification of sexual dysfunctions: Towards DSM-V and ICD–11. Comprehensive Psychiatry: 39(6) 333–337, 1998

Whipple B: Women's sexual pleasure and satisfaction: a new view of female sexual function. Female Patient, 27, 39–44, 2001

## 2

# The Biopsychosocial Evaluation and Treatment of Sexual Disorders

WAGUIH WILLIAM ISHAK, M.D.

## I. Introduction

The Biopsychosocial model began early in the 20th century by psychiatrist Adolf Meyer and was most clearly articulated by George Engel (Engel 1980). Using insights from general systems theory, developed by the biologists Ludwig von Bertalanffy and Paul Weiss, Engel argued that mental disorders occur within individuals who are part of a whole system. This system has sub-personal (nervous system, cells, molecules) and supra-personal (relationships, community, society) elements. Attempts of explaining and treating mental disorders using only sub-personal elements (what some call biological or biomedical) carry the risk of reductionism and inadequacy to explain and address supra-personal elements that are essential for the human experience.

Unlike other disorders of bodily functions, sexual behavior almost always involves a partner in reality or in fantasy. The theme of "it takes two" had seemed to be minimized in current clinical practice especially after the revolutionary developments in biological interventions (namely oral PhosphoDiEstrase–5 inhibitors). Hence, it is crucial to utilize the Biopsychosocial approach in evaluating and treating sexual disorders by engaging both partners and, examining and addressing both the cause and effect on the relationship.

## II. The Biopsychosocial Evaluation

A. **Definition:** This type of evaluation comprises evaluating the individuals and the couple aiming at identifying predisposing, precipitating, and perpetuating factors of sexual dysfunction:

1. Evaluation of the Individuals:
   a. Biological factors:
      1) Genetic predisposition
      2) Medical problems
      3) Substance effects
   b. Psychosocial factors:
      1) Psychiatric disorders
      2) Traumas, losses, and conflicts
      3) Financial, vocational, and residential factors
2. Evaluation of the Couple:
   a. Sexual knowledge, skills, and attitude
   b. Relationship, commitment, and motivation

B. **Biological Factors Affecting Sexual Functioning**

1. Genetic predisposition: Most of the genetic studies in this field focused on sexual orientation. Bailey and Pillard (1991) studied a sample of gay men including identical and fraternal twins, non-twin biological brothers and unrelated adopted brothers. The concordance rate for identical twins was 52 percent, for the fraternal twins it was 22 percent, non-twin biological brothers was 9 percent, and adopted brothers was 11 percent. In sexual disorders,

Waldinger et al. (1998) reported cases of familial occurrence of premature ejaculation while Fischer et al. (2004) concluded that the estimated heritability of liability for dysfunction in having an erection is 35% and in maintaining an erection is 42%. Apart from medical conditions caused by hereditary factors that could lead to sexual dysfunction, genetic predisposition to sexual disorders is largely a poorly studied issue.

2. Medical problems:

a. Systemic disease: Diabetes Mellitus, anemia, hypertension, hyperlipidemia, heart disease, atherosclerosis, aneurysms, smoking, and poor diet habits, are etiologically related to sexual disorders.

b. Hormonal and endocrinal: Hypothyroidism or hyperthyroidism, hypothalamic/pituitary axis dysregulation (manifested by high or low hormonal levels), hypogonadism, pituitary tumors, surgical removal of gonads, natural or surgical menopause, and ovarian failure.

c. Neurological spinal cord injury, disease of the central or peripheral nervous system, including diabetes and peripheral neuropathy.

d. Medical illnesses that limit physical activity such as arthritis and cardiac problems need to be also evaluated.

e. Genital disease: congenital abnormalities, blunt trauma, peyronie's disease (scarring on the penile dorsum), pelvic fractures, post-surgical, and in women extensive bike riding, was reported to result in diminished vaginal and clitoral blood flow

3. Substance effects: The impact of different substances and medications on sexual functioning is detailed in Chapter 3 and also in the etiology section in on sexual desire, arousal, orgasm, and pain disorders.

## C. Psychosocial Factors Affecting Sexual Functioning of the Individual

1. Psychiatric disorders: Psychotic, Mood, Anxiety, and Somatoform Disorders all could lead to sexual dysfunction (see Appendix 3). For

more details on the impact of specific psychiatric disorders on sexual functioning, please review the etiology section in chapters on sexual desire, arousal, orgasm, and pain disorders.

2. Traumas, losses, and conflicts, in addition to financial, vocational, and residential factors all interfere with the three phases of the Sexual Response Cycle and might be underlying Sexual Pain Disorders.

## D. Psychosocial Factors Affecting Sexual Functioning of the Couple

1. Sexual knowledge, skills, and attitude: Impairment in knowledge, deficient skills, and poor attitude could negatively affect sexual functioning. Knowledge about the anatomy, and physiology of sexual organs generally start in school as sex education (for prevention of sexually transmitted disease, early pregnancy, abortion) in a standard part of basic education in many countries around the world. The need for ongoing education cannot be overemphasized. However, sexual skills are generally not addressed except during treatment of sexual disorders. Fortunately, a plethora of sexual enhancement non-pornographic books and videos that exists in this era is extremely helpful. Attitude towards sex is a very complicated issue that encompasses issues from the past such as upbringing, issues from the present such as fear of pregnancy, and issues from the future such as relationship prospectives.

2. Relationship, commitment, and motivation: A thorough evaluation of the current relationship is crucial is determining the underlying factors leading to sexual dysfunction in the couple. Grossly conflictual, ambivalent, and distant relationships are some of the more commonly seen model of relationships associated with sexual problems. Genograms are particularly helpful to explain how patterns of family communication are transmitted from one generation to another. Another important issue to evaluate with the couple is their commitment and motivation to ameliorate the sexual problem. Partners who are engaged in extra-relational sexual activities or those who are no longer interested in their partner should not be enrolled in sex therapy but should be referred for couple therapy work in order to clarify these issues.

From a practical point of view confidentiality of each partner still needs to be protected.

**E. Biopsychosocial Evaluation Procedure:**

1. Establishing rapport remains the most important factors in any psychiatric or medical evaluation. Empathy, genuine concern and professional style are the basic components of establishing effective rapport with patients experiencing sexual problems who would be understandably reluctant to discuss sexual issues in clinical settings. JAMA reported a telephone survey of 500 patients prepared by a public opinion research firm revealing that 71% of patients thought their doctor would dismiss concerns they would bring up about sexual problems, and 68% were afraid of embarrassing their physicians by discussing sexual dysfunction (Marwick 1999).

2. Sexual history

   Collecting information about the Chief Complaint, History of Present Illness (HPI), Past Sexual Disorders History, Personal Sexual History, Psychiatric History, Substance Use History and Medical History are all essential elements of the Biopsychosocial evaluation of patients with sexual disorders.

   a. The setting:

   Sexual history is collected in extremely variable settings: during routine medical check up, visits to family practitioners, primary care physicians, internists, gynecologists and obstetricians, urologists, cardiologists, adolescent medicine specialists, infectious disease specialists, emergency physicians, psychiatrists, couple therapists, individual therapists, nutritionists, nurses, clergy, and even legal practitioners. Another setting variables include individual evaluation versus couple evaluation, or adolescents' interviews witnessed by their parents. The Association of Reproductive Health Professionals recommended that a third party be present during sexual history taking if a patient is impaired, litigious, acts or speaks in a sexual manner. In the mental health field, ideally the couple would be evaluated together initially then individually, followed by another couple meeting.

b. The opening:

Obstacles to collecting a relevant sexual history include patient-based factors such as embarrassment, talking in front of a partner, clinician-based factors such as discomfort with the subject, awkwardness with language, fear of offending the patient and system-based factors such as confidentiality, documentation of details in medical records, and legal risks. It is very important for clinicians to be sensitive, direct, clear, detail-oriented, to modulate own reactions, and to alleviate patient's misperceptions of perversions or abnormality. It is also important for clinicians not to ask questions out of mere curiosity, make assumptions or judgments or obviously share personal experiences (Sadock et al. 1997, IsHak et al. 2005). Floyd et al. (1999) studied interviewing techniques for sexual practices and used the following questions to introduce exploration of sexual problems in a primary care setting:

- "You've told me about your lifestyle, your occupation, exercise, and diet. Now I'm going to ask you some questions about your sexual activities" helps the transition to sexual history (lifestyle bridge).
- "I routinely ask all my patients about their sexual history...I'm now going to ask you some questions about your sexual activities" makes collecting this information part of the normal procedure for this physician (ubiquity statement).
- "How do you feel about answering some questions about your sexual activity?" elicits feelings about exploring this area.
- "I'm now going to ask you about your sexual activities" is a direct approach to collecting sexual history (direct statement)
- "Please describe your sexual activities" is an open-ended question about sexual practices.
- "Are you currently sexually active with a partner" is a closed-ended question about sexual activity.

Although more studies are needed to explore the patient comfort in relation to gender or sexual orientation (explicit) of the clinician, in the above study, participants expressed more comfort with transition with statistically insignificant favoring the ubiquity statement over the lifestyle bridge. Gender differences were also explored and revealed that men were more comfortable when the direct statement method was used and women felt more comfortable with closed-ended questions compared to men (Floyd et al. 1999). Pomeroy (1982) recommended the use of 'gentle assumption' where in a gentle voice; questions are framed along the lines of "how frequently do you find yourself masturbating, if at all?" rather than "do you masturbate?" leading to more revealing answers about potentially embarrassing behaviors. Non-verbal communication could be more utilized by clinicians during sexual history interviews (Tomlinson 1998). Depending on the gender of the patient, it would be important to utilize transitional, feelings-eliciting, direct, open-ended, and closed-ended questions in order to maximize the outcome. Structured interviewing have been also used in clinics specialized in the evaluation and treatment of sexual disorders.

c.  Chief Complaint and History of Present Illness (HPI)

If sexual problems are identified it is crucial to establish a clear Chief Sexual Complaint and HPI before proceeding to collect the rest of the sexual history. A Chief Sexual Complaint has to be identified as occurring in one of the three phases of the Sexual Response Cycle (Desire, Arousal, Orgasm), or is related to Pain. The HPI would aim at identifying the onset, course, duration (lifetime or acquired), associated symptoms and signs, impact on functioning, precipitating factors (generalized or situational), and whether dysfunction is occurring in the context of an identified general medical condition or substance intake (due to psychological or combined factors).

d.  Past sexual disorders history: understanding whether the past history of the same or different disorders help shed some light on lifetime or acquired disorders in addition to generalized or situational ones. Examining past history of response to different interventions is also of value to the evaluating clinician.

e.  Family history of sexual disorders: very little is known about genetic factors in sexual disorders.

f. Personal sexual history: there has been a debate over how much exploration needs to be done in this area. Most clinicians tend to obtain a chronological account of early sexual activities, puberty, sexual orientation issues, masturbatory practices, sexual relationships, pregnancy, abortion, sexual assaults, ageing effects, menopause, current relationship details, frequency of sexual activity, preferred sexual practices, and satisfaction level. Important points include medical high-risk behaviors e.g., sexually transmitted diseases, history of sexual abuse, and unlawful practices such as pedophilia.

g. Psychiatric history: psychiatric disorders could lead to a variety of sexual disorders. It is important to rule out (or detect) Disorders Dating Since Childhood such as Autism, Psychotic disorders such as Schizophrenia, Mood disorders such as Major Depressive Disorder, Anxiety disorders such as Panic Disorder, Somatoform Disorders such as Pain Disorder, Eating Disorders such as Anorexia, and Personality Disorders.

h. Substance use history: substances include alcohol, illicit drugs, prescription and over the counter medications, herbal and dietary supplements and toxins. Sexual symptoms developed during, or within a month of, Substance Intoxication or medication use that is deemed etiologically related to sexual dysfunction should raise suspicion about the presence of a Substance-Induced Sexual Dysfunction (APA 2000).

i. Medical history: in addition history of medical and surgical problems, a review of the following systems is necessary to complete a sexual dysfunction evaluation: Constitutional Symptoms (usual weight and recent change, weakness, fever, chills, night sweats, fatigue, malaise, hot/cold intolerance, change in appetite), Skin, Head, Eyes, Ears, Nose, Throat, Respiratory, Cardiac, Breasts, Gastrointestinal, Genitourinary, Neurological, Musculoskeletal, Hematological, and Endocrinal systems. More emphasis is needed on vascular, genital, neurological, endocrinological, and operative issues.

3. Physical exam: a detailed and thorough physical exam that includes all systems mentioned in the review of systems should cover:

General appearance, Vital signs, Skin, hair, nails, Head, Eyes, Ears, Nose, Mouth, Neck, Chest, Heart, Breasts, Abdomen, Extremities, Neurological exam, Genitalia rectum and prostate (male), and Pelvic exam (females). More emphasis is needed on secondary sexual characteristics, abdominal examination (aneurysms), major pulse examination (atherosclerosis), neurological assessment, and external genitalia/pelvic examination. For more details on the specific impact of medical disorders on sexual functioning, please review the etiology section in chapters on sexual desire, arousal, orgasm, and pain disorders.

4. Psychiatric exam: a detailed and thorough mental status exam should be performed to clarify some findings obtained through the Psychiatric history. A crucial issue for this item in sexual disorders is the assessment of the level of sexual knowledge, skills, and attitude. In examining a couple, this is the time to assess the current relationship, commitment, and motivation for sexual behavior and satisfaction.

5. Assessment instruments: Arizona Sexual Experiences Scale (McGahuey et al. 1998), the Changes in Sexual Functioning Questionnaire, clinical version (Clayton et al. 1997), and the International Index Of Erectile Function (IIEF) (Rosen et al. 1999). This writer co-authored web-based assessment instruments in 1997, to enable users in the privacy of their own locale to get an initial screening about the presence of sexual symptoms warranting a psychiatric or a medical evaluation. Please review on the New York University School of Medicine Department of Psychiatry website: Online Sexual Disorders Screening for Women at http://www.med.nyu.edu/Psych/screens/sdsf.html and the Online Sexual Disorders Screening for Men at http://www.med.nyu.edu/Psych/screens/sdsm.html. Copies of the screening tests are included in Appendix II. More specific instruments are recommended in the respective chapters.

6. Laboratory investigations:

   a. Standard labs: complete metabolic panels, complete blood count, lipid profiles, urine analysis, thyroid function tests, kidney function tests, liver function tests, and hormonal levels are standard in sexual disorders evaluation.

b. Hormonal levels are an essential part of the evaluation although normal ranges are still debated and depend on laboratory methods and lack of established norms. Hormonal levels include Luteinizing Hormone (LH) normal = 5–15 mIU/mL, Follicle-Stimulating Hormone (FSH) (normal = 5–15 mIU/mL), Prolactin (normal <15 mIU/mL), Total Testosterone (normal= 300–1,000 ng/dL in adult males and 30–120 ng/dL in adult females), Free Testosterone (normal using the equilibrium ultrafiltration method=5.00–21.00 ng/dL in adult males and 0.3–0.85 ng/dL in adult females). Serum for testosterone measurement should be drawn between 8:00 A.M. and 10:00 A.M., and not during the early follicular phase in premenopausal women. Sex hormone-binding globulin (SHBG) is the specific plasma transport protein for sex steroid hormones (dihydrotestosterone, testosterone, and estradiol) in humans. Normal values are 0.6–3.5 mg/L in adult men and 2.5–5.4 mg/L in adult nonpregnant women. Caution needs to be exercised in interpreting hormonal level results as they are affected by a number of factors including medical or physiological conditions, diet, and stress.

c. Nocturnal penile tumescence and rigidity analysis.

d. Direct injection of Prostaglandin $E_1$ ($PGE_1$) into the penis, a medication that increases blood flow into the penis and normally produces erections. If the penile structure is normal or at least adequate, an erection should develop within several minutes.

e. Vascular testing such as duplex ultrasound and dynamic infusion: cavernosometry and cavernosography.

f. Neurological testing such as a biothesiometry (measuring sensory perception threshold of the penis or female genital points), somatosensory evoked potentials and pudendal electromyography.

g. Newer investigations for women include techniques developed by the Berman Sisters at Boston University and later at UCLA including: pH probes to measure lubrication; a balloon device to evaluate the ability of the vagina to relax and dilate; vibratory and heat and cold sensation measures of the external and internal genitalia; and high frequency Doppler imaging, or ultrasound, to measure blood flow to the vagina and clitoris during arousal (Berman 2003).

h. Measurement of vaginal and minor labial oxygen tension using a modified Clark oxygen electrode to obtain partial oxygen pressure (pO$_2$) (Sommer et al 2001).

7. Formulation and diagnosis

The Biopsychosocial formulation will contain the following elements:

- Identifying information
- Target sexual symptoms and signs
- Biological factors of the individuals (medical problems, or substance effects)
- Psychosocial factors of the individuals (psychiatric disorders, traumas, losses, and conflicts, financial, vocational, and residential problems)
- Psychosocial factors of the couple (sexual knowledge, skills, and attitude, relationship, commitment, and motivation)

At this point, three very important diagnoses will need to be ruled out or detected for further evaluation and treatment.

a. An Axis I Psychiatric Disorder that better accounts for the sexual disorder.

b. A Substance-Induced Sexual Dysfunction (see Chapter 3 for more details)

c. A Sexual Dysfunction Due to a General Medical Condition (See Chapter 4 for more details)

The remaining diagnoses according to the DSM-IV-TR are:

a. Sexual Desire Disorders (men and women):

1) Sexual Aversion Disorder

2) Hypoactive Sexual Desire Disorder

b. Sexual Arousal Disorders:

1) Female Sexual Arousal Disorder

2) Male Erectile Disorder

   c. Orgasmic Disorders:

     1) Female Orgasmic Disorder

     2) Male Orgasmic Disorder

     3) Premature Ejaculation

   d. Sexual Pain Disorders:

     1) Dyspareunia

     2) Vaginismus

   e. It is important to specify whether the above disorders are:

     1) Lifelong type or acquired type

     2) Generalized type or situational type

     3) Due to psychological factors or due to combined factors

   f. Sexual Dysfunction NOS (302.70): the sexual disorder does not meet the criteria of any specific disorder within this category.

## III. The Biopsychosocial Treatment Plan

A comprehensive Biopsychosocial plan takes into account interventions that address all the factors involved in predisposing, precipitating or perpetuating the sexual disorder.

### A. Biological Interventions:

1. General medical conditions: it is essential to treat endocrinal abnormalities such as hypothyroidism, correct hormonal deficiencies such as low testosterone, and manage physically-limiting disorders such as arthritis.

2. Substance-Induced Sexual Disorders: identifying and replacing (or discontinuing) agents responsible for sexual disorders is the definitive treatment in many situations where sexual functioning could be ameliorated. For more details on the treatment of substance-induced sexual disorders, especially SSRI-induced sexual dysfunction, the reader is referred to Chapter 3.

3. Administer oral medications (Phosphodiestrase–5 inhibitors, non PDE–5 agents, antidepressants, hormones), injections, pellets, implants, or devices.

 We will provide here details about Phosphodiestrase–5, injections, pellets, implants, and devices.

 a. Phosphodiestrase–5 inhibitors (PDE–5 Inhibitors): Phosphodiesterase (PDE) is an enzyme that causes breakdown of cyclic GMP, which is the direct intracellular mediator in the nitric oxide (nonadrenergic, noncholinergic) pathway. The nitric oxide system causes relaxation of smooth muscle in blood vessel walls, i.e., vasodilatation, in various organ systems. PDE catalyzes the degradation of cGMP. Type 5 PDE is concentrated in the penile smooth muscle of the corpus cavernosum, and by inhibiting PDE–5; less cGMP is degraded leading to continued vasodilatation and promotion of erection. Sildenafil (Viagra), Vardenafil (Levitra) and Tadalfil (Cialis) all inhibit PDE–5 leading to erection and maintenance of erection in response to sexual stimulation.

 1) Sildenafil (Viagra)

 | | |
 |---|---|
 | Effectiveness: | A recent report by Steers et al analyzing the data from several studies demonstrated that sildenafil provided long-term satisfaction for the majority of patients: 36-week study: 269 patients (80%) completed treatment, median duration of therapy was 252 days. 92% of patients reported improved erections at end of study. 52-week studies (3): 565 patients (84%) completed treatment; mean duration of therapy was 358 days. 87% of patients reported improved erections at end of studies. |
 | Common Side effects: | Headache, Flushing, Dyspepsia and Nasal Congestion. |
 | Drug Interactions: | Nitrates, alpha-blockers and protease inhibitors. |
 | Dosing: | 25 mg, 50 mg, and 100 mg. For most men, the recommended starting dose is 50 mg/day one to four hours before intercourse. |

 2) Vardenafil (Levitra)

 | | |
 |---|---|
 | Effectiveness: | A study of over 800 men with ED showed: 74% of men taking a 20 mg dose of Levitra and 77% taking a 10 mg dose were able to have intercourse on their first attempt, compared with 45% taking a placebo. |

|  |  |
|---|---|
| | Those men receiving treatment who were successful the first time continued to achieve successful penetration in 91% of their subsequent attempts. |
| Side effects: | Those involved in the clinical trials reported mild/moderate side effects with the treatment, these mostly included headaches, flushing and rhinitis (nasal congestion). |
| Drug Interactions: | Nitrates, Alpha-blockers: Hytrin® (terazosin HCl), Flomax® (tamsulosin HCl), Cardura® (doxazosin mesylate), Minipress® (prazosin HCl) or Uroxatral® (alfuzosin HCl). Antiarrhythmics. These include quinidine, procainamide, amiodarone and sotalol. Protease Inhbitors: ritonavir (Norvir®) or indinavir sulfate (Crixivan®). Antifungals: ketoconazole or itraconazole (such as Nizoral® or Sporanox®). Erythromycin and other erectile dysfunction treatments. |
| Dosing: | 2.5 mg, 5 mg, 10 mg, and 20 mg. For most men, the recommended starting dose is 10 mg/day one to four hours before intercourse. |

## 3) Tadalafil (Cialis)

|  |  |
|---|---|
| Effectiveness: | A recent clinical study on nearly 400 men with ED. The study was designed to evaluate the efficiency of Cialis 10–20mg at specific time points after dosing (24 or 36 hours). 88 percent of men achieved erections in 30 minutes or less, it continued to stay in the system for up to 24 hours, in secondary measures of efficacy—including the ability to penetrate, satisfaction with hardness of erection and overall satisfaction, it was superior to the placebo at both 24 and 36 hours. |
| Side effects: | Headaches, dyspepsia, flushing, back pain and muscle aches (pains are usually 12 to 24 hours after taking the medication). |
| Drug Interactions: | Nitrates, Alpha-blockers except Flomax® (tamsulosin HCl), (These include Hytrin® (terazosin HCl), Cardura® (doxazosin mesylate), Minipress® (prazosin HCl) or Uroxatral® (alfuzosin HCl). ritonavir (Norvir®) or indinavir (Crixivan®) ketoconazole or itraconazole (such as Nizoral® or Sporanox®). Erythromycin and other erectile dysfunction treatments. |
| Dosing: | 5 mg, 10 mg, and 20 mg. For most men, the recommended starting dose is 10 mg/day not necessarily before intercourse. |

Details on the use of the three medications (including differences) in Male Erectile Disorder are presented in Chapter 6 on Sexual Arousal Disorders.

b. Injection therapy typically uses a combination of drugs prescribed by (usually) a urologist. The man directly injects the drugs into the side of his penis. The drugs relax muscles and increase blood flow to create an erection. The most common drugs are Papavarine, Phentolamine and alprostadil. The MD may combine two or all three of these drugs. The drugs are injected directly into the penis through a fine-gauge "insulin-style" needle. A firm erection develops in 10–15 minutes and lasts up to 60 minutes.

c. Pellets

The most common urethral suppositories are known as MUSE®, which stands for "medicated urethral system for erection." The drug in MUSE is alprostadil. A man generally will get an erection within 10–15 minutes of application. The erection will last about 30–60 minutes. MUSE works for only about 30% of men who try it. Sometimes MUSE provides only a partial erection. Some men will then use penile injection or a vacuum erection device to attain a complete erection.

d. Implants: the most advanced is the Three-piece inflatable penile implant. Most closely resembles the process and "feel" of a natural erection. More details are provided in Chapter 6 on Sexual Arousal Disorders.

e. Devices: Vacuum devices for both men and women to enhance erection (men) and clitoral sensation and arousal (women).

## B. Psychosocial interventions:

1. Sex therapy:

Originally developed by Masters and Johnson sex therapy is a psychosocial therapy that focuses on the sexual relationship of the couple involving increased awareness of pleasurable body sensations exercises named collectively Sensate focus. Sensate focus is a series of specific exercises for couples, which encourages each partner to take turns paying increased attention to their own senses.

In the first stage, the couple takes turns touching each other's body, excluding the breasts and genitals. The purpose of the touching is not necessary sexual but to heighten awareness of sensations while touching or being touched by the partner. There is no particular order or expectations of what would please the partner. This the process by which each of the partners will learn more in depth about these issues when they process the exercises in their next therapist appointment. The couple is prohibited from having intercourse, if sexual arousal does occur; they are instructed to masturbate individually afterwards if the urge cannot be resisted. Masters and Johnson recommended silence so that couple could focus on physical sensations.

Sensate focus II is the following stage where the breasts and genitals are now included (and not focused on or started with) in the pleasurable touching routines. The couple learns through meeting with their therapist about their heightened physical sensation awareness, their 'hot spots' and they will learn new techniques such as 'hand guiding'. By having one hand on top of the partner's hand while being touched, the partner could communicate non-verbally regarding more or less pressure, a faster or slower pace, or a change to a different spot.

In the next phase of sensate focus, mutual touching is introduced, and as the couple progresses genito-genital touch is added using the female-on-top position without attempting insertion of the penis into the vagina. For heterosexual couples, the penis (regardless the state of erection) is rubbed against the vulva, clitoris, and vaginal opening. As the couple is more comfortable with more intense contacts without rushing into sexual intercourse (which remains prohibited), insertion of a semi-erected penis could be tried with moving to non-genital touching if arousal becomes too intense and orgasm is impending. More sessions of this level would be processed with the therapist and then the couple is allowed to have full intercourse.

2. Couple therapy:

Couple therapy helps define more clearly the issues between partners in a couple, develop more insights into the dynamics of their relationship and helps enhance communication.

It is designed for unmarried or married couples, couples contemplating marriage or for couples dealing with various life adjustment situations (career change, children, or moving, etc.). Behavioral techniques such as 'active listening', 'talking and listening exercises', 'assertiveness training', 'role playing', are utilized depending on the type of couple therapy. Types of couple therapy include: Brief Strategic, Cognitive-Behavioral, Object Relations, Structural–Strategic, Transgenerational, Affective Reconstructive, Emotionally Focused, Collaborative, Narrative, Solution-Focused, and Integrative Couple Therapy. For more details please review Gurman and Jacobson (2002).

3. Individual psychotherapy

Individual psychotherapy helps define more clearly the issues within the individual, develop more insights into the dynamics of relating and helps enhance coping skills. Types of individual therapy include: Supportive, Psychodynamic or psychoanalytic, Cognitive-Behavioral, Behavioral, and Interpersonal Psychotherapy.

4. Group psychotherapy

Sexual disorders are not usually discussed in group settings but group psychotherapy is most useful for patients coping with life stressors or traumas, patients with psychiatric disorders, patients with co-morbid medical conditions or substance abuse.

5. Social work consultations, financial, and vocational counseling

It is essential for treatment success that patients are offered interventions designed to address their significant concerns such as money, living situations, career problems. Access to Social work consultations, financial, and vocational counseling is important in this regard.

## C. Other Interventions

1. Aphrodisiacs

Aphrodisiacs are substances that arouse sexual desire or enhance sexual performance. Among the many substances that have been claimed to have such an effect are oysters, ginseng root, powdered rhinoceros horn, animal testicles, and turtles' eggs. The effectiveness of the so-called aphrodisiacs is largely unknown and could be seriously questionable given the fact the placebo-response rate in sexual research amounts to about 50%. Information on alternative medicine approaches for sexual enhancement is discussed in details in Chapter 9.

2. Sexual positions:

The most common sexual positions are man-on-top, woman-on-top, side-by-side, and rear-entry. They may all be modified by performing them lying down, sitting, standing, kneeling, or any combination of these. It is not really clear if there are certain positions that are more sexually enhancing than others, however, most couples seen in clinical settings agree that a variety of positions adds more satisfaction to sexual experiences. The one position that could be singled out in this regard for heterosexuals would be the rear-entry (or sometimes side entry) for its stimulation of anterior vaginal wall leading to a possible stimulation of the Grafenberg spot (G-spot). Some women report more intense orgasms related to this stimulation.

3. Sex surrogates:

Masters and Johnson introduced sex surrogate therapy as a highly effective therapeutic modality for single men (Masters and Johnson 1970). Surrogates are regulated by a code of conduct by the International Professional Surrogates Association (IPSA). Perhaps the most significant study about surrogacy was performed by Noonan (1984) in the course of his master's degree at New York University. The study demonstrated according to the author that almost 90% of the surrogate's time is spent in non-sexual activities: 48.5% in experiential, non-erotic exercises: 34% in talking, giving sex information and emotional support and reassurance; and 5% focusing on social skills in public settings, and only 13% of the surrogate's time is spent engaging in sexual activities. Sexual surrogacy remains in the center of a complex moral, ethical and professional dilemma and is usually not recommended by practicing sex therapists.

## IV. Outcome Assessment, Re-evaluation, and Re-planning

It is important to use valid and reliable measures periodically to assess the outcome of treatment interventions. The most common instruments used for outcome assessment in this field are highlighted in Table 1 (Berman et al. 2002) provided extensive details on these outcome measures.

This author recommends outcome assessment and re-evaluation every three months in order to detect response, partial response, or lack of response. Patients who are not responding will need a thorough re-evaluation using the guidelines mentioned before. Treatment re-planning is a necessity once more factors for treatment response problems have been identified.

| TABLE 1 Outcome Measures of Sexual Disorders | | |
|---|---|---|
| **Category** | **Measurement** | |
| **General Global Sexual Functioning** | Sexual History Form (SHF) | Deragotis Sexual Function Inventory (DSFI) | Sexual Interaction Inventory (SII) |
| **Male Gender Specific Global Sexual Functioning** | Erectile Dysfunction Inventory of Tx. Satis. (EDITS) | Brief Male Sexual Function Inventory for Urology | Gender Identity and Erotic Preferences in Males |
| **Female Gender Specific Global Sexual Functioning** | McCoy Female Sexuality Questionnaire (MFSQ) | Brief Index for Sexual Functioning (BISF-W) | Female Sexual Arousal Index (FSAI) |
| **Sexual Self Concept** | Multidimensional Sexual Self-Concept Ques. (MSSCQ) | Sexual Self Efficacy Scale Erectile Functioning (SSES-E) | Sexual Self-Efficacy Scale for Female Functioning (SSES-F) |
| **Relationship Measures** | Index of Sexual Satisfaction (ISS) | Sexual Interaction System Scale (SISS) | Sexual Relationship Scale (SRS) |

Reprinted with permission from Berman et al.: Outcome Measurement in Sexual Disorders, in IsHak WW, Burt T, Sederer LI (Editors) Outcome Measurement in Psychiatry: A Critical Review, American Psychiatric Press, Washington DC, 2002

## V. Conclusion

The Biopsychosocial evaluation and treatment of sexual disorders involves engaging both partners in addressing the sexual problem and examining thoroughly all the factors that might contribute to its generation. These factors include biological ones (genetic, substance-induced, medical illness), and psychosocial ones (psychiatric disorders, stressors, and relationship issues). The treatment should address:

A. **The Individuals** (for clinician from all specialties sharing sexual disorders)

1. Treatment of the underlying etiology of Sexual Disorders due to General Medical Conditions and Substance-Induced Sexual Disorders including treatment of hormonal deficiencies, and medication-induced disorders.

2. Evaluate/administer medications, injections, pellets, implants, or devices.

3. Treatment of psychiatric symptoms and disorders (Psychotic, Mood, Anxiety, Somatoform, and other disorders).

4. Treatment of psychosocial factors (traumas, losses, conflicts) using individual or group psychotherapy.

5. Addressing residential, vocational, and financial problems using social work, career and financial counseling.

B. **The Couple** (for mental health professionals)

1. Sex education utilizing educational illustrations, books, and videos.

2. Sex therapy

## *References*

American Psychiatric Association (APA): Diagnostic and Statistical Manual of Mental Disorders. 4th ed. Text Revision. Washington, DC, American Psychiatric Publishing Inc, 2000

Bailey JM, Pillard R: A Genetic Study of Male Sexual Orientation. Archives of General Psychiatry 48: 1089–96, 1991

Berman L, Berman J, Zierak MC, Marley C: Outcome Measurement in Sexual Disorders, in IsHak WW, Burt T, Sederer LI (Editors) Outcome Measurement in Psychiatry: A Critical Review. Washington DC, American Psychiatric Press, 2002

Berman J and Berman L: http://www.urology.medsch.ucla.edu/fsmc_home.html, 2003

Clayton AH, McGarvey EL, Clavet GJ: The Changes in Sexual Functioning Questionnaire (CSFQ): development, reliability, and validity. Psychopharmacol Bull. 33:731–745, 1997

Engel GL: The clinical application of the biopsychosocial model. American Journal of Psychiatry 137: 535–544, 1980

Fischer ME, Vitek ME, Hedeker D, et al.: A twin study of erectile dysfunction. Archives of Internal Medicine 164(2):165–8, 2004

Floyd M. Lang F. Beine KL. McCord E: Evaluating interviewing techniques for the sexual practices history. Use of video trigger tapes to assess patient comfort. Archives of Family Medicine 8(3):218–23, 1999

Gurman AS and Jacobson NS (Editors): Clinical Handbook of Couple Therapy, Third Edition. New York, NY, Guilford Publications, 2002

Hajos M, Fleishaker JC, Filipiak-Reisner JK, et al: The selective norepinephrine reuptake inhibitor antidepressant reboxetine: pharmacological and clinical profile. CNS Drug Rev.10(1):23–44, 2004

IsHak WW, Amiri SR, and Michaeli D: Sexual History: The Art and the Science. Presented at the annual meeting of the American Psychiatric Association, Atlanta, May 2005

Marwick C: Survey says patients expect little physician help on sex. JAMA. 281(23):2173–4, 1999

Masters, W and Johnson, V: Human sexual inadequacy. Boston, MA, Little, Brown, 1970, pp 146–156

McGahuey CA, Gelenberg AJ, Laukes CA, et al.: The Arizona Sexual Experiences Scale (ASEX): reliability and validity. J Sex Marital Ther. 26:25–40, 1998

Noonan, RJ: Sex surrogates: A clarification of their functions. http://www.SexQuest.com/surrogat.htm. New York: SexQuest/The Sex Institute, 1984

Pomeroy WB: Taking a sex history: interviewing and recording. New York, NY, Free Press, 1982

Rosen RC, Cappelleri JC, Smith MD, Lipsky J Pena BM: Development and evaluation of an abridged, 5-item version of the International Index of Erectile Function (IIEF–5) as a diagnostic tool for erectile dysfunction. International Journal of Impotence Research 11: 319–26, 1999

Sadock VA, IsHak WW, and Michaeli D: How much do we know about our patients' sexual history? Presented at the annual meeting of the American Psychiatric Association, San Diego, May 1997

Sadock VA: Normal Human Sexuality and Sexual Dysfunctions. In Sadock VA and Sadock BJ (Eds.) Comprehensive Textbook of Psychiatry. Baltimore, MD, Lippincott Williams & Wilkins Publishers, 7th edition 2000, pp 1577–1608

Sommer F, Caspers HP, Esders K, et al.: Measurement of vaginal and minor labial oxygen tension for the evaluation of female sexual function. Journal of Urology 165(4):1181–4, 2001

Tomlinson J: Taking a Sexual History. http://bmj.bmjjournals.com/cgi/reprint/317/7172/1573.pdf BMJ 317:15736, 1998

Waldinger MD, Rietschel M., Nothen MM, Hengeveld, MW and Olivier B: Familial occurrence of primary premature ejaculation. Psychiatr Genet 8: 37, 1998

# 3

# Substance-Induced Sexual Dysfunction

WAGUIH WILLIAM ISHAK, M.D.
STEPHANIE MICHAEL STEWART, M.D.
ROBERT N. PECHNICK, PH.D.
WILLIAM HUANG, M.D.
ERNST R. SCHWARZ, M.D., PH.D.

## I. Introduction

Modern understanding of the neurobiochemical mechanisms underlying sexual behavior has evolved over the last few decades. Breakthrough discoveries were made in understanding local (genital) mechanisms while more developments in understanding central nervous system mechanisms are underway. Part of the work that earned Louis Ignarro, Ph.D. the Nobel Prize in Medicine in 1998 had significantly impacted the lives of millions of people worldwide. The discovery of the role of nitric oxide as a mediator for relaxation of the corpus cavernosum (Rajfer, Aronson, Bush, Dorey, and Ignarro 1992) lead to the production of sildenafil, the first medication to effectively treat erectile dysfunction, that was approved by the U.S. Food And Drug Administration (FDA) in March of 1998 and is marketed since then. Further research is still needed to define the neurotransmitters responsible for vaginal smooth muscle relaxation, the role of sex steroid hormones and their receptors in modulating genital hemodynamics, smooth muscle contractility and neurotransmitter receptor expression. A global and integral understanding of the biologic aspects of sexual function requires investigation of the vascular, neurological (central and peripheral) and structural components of this extremely complex physiological process. Knowledge of the effects of substances on sexual dysfunction helps us understand the mechanisms of normal sexual behavior. This chapter will review the effects of neurotransmitters, hormones, and substances causing sexual dysfunction as well as some proposed treatment strategies.

## II. Effects of Neurotransmitters and Hormones on Sexual Behavior

### A. Serotonin

Elevated serotonin levels generally inhibit sexual behavior; however antagonism of serotonin postsynaptic receptor subtypes can either enhance or block the effect of serotonin on sexual functioning. In female rats, 5-HT$_{1A}$ and 5-HT$_3$ receptors inhibit lordosis (a receptive sexual behavior in rats), while 5-HT$_{1B}$, 5-HT$_{1C}$, or 5-HT$_2$ receptors facilitate lordosis. Direct agonist in other subtypes can enhance sexual behavior. In male rats, a selective 5-HT$_{1A}$ receptor agonist markedly increased sexual behavior, leading to ejaculation after only one or two intromissions, rather than the usual ten to twelve intromissions (Pfaus 1999). Coordination of other neurotransmitter pathways is also essential, as serotonin is only one of the many neurotransmitters involved in sexual functioning.

### B. Norepinephrine

Adrenergic receptors have been shown to be present in the brain and spinal cord of animals and humans. Animal studies suggest that central adrenergic activation lead to an increase sexual behavior, which would account for the ameliorative effects of dextroamphetamine and pemoline (sympathomimetics), as well as yohimbine (an alpha–2 adrenergic receptor antagonist). In female rats, stimulation of alpha–1 receptors in the ventromedial nucleus of the hypothalamus (VMH) plays a role in the hormonal facilitation of lordosis behavior, while stimulation of beta-receptors in the preoptic area appears to inhibit lordosis (Pfaus 1999). Locally, beta-adrenergic receptors facilitate the increase in blood flow into sinuses, while alpha-adrenergic receptors facilitate the termination of erection via a direct constrictor effect on musculature. Additionally, cholinergic receptors are thought to modulate adrenergic activity for optimal sexual functioning, but do not seem to act directly.

## C. Dopamine

Increased central dopaminergic activity also appears to increase sexual behavior and functioning. Apomorphine, a mixed D1 and D2 dopamine receptor agonist, increases the likelihood of spontaneous erections in normal volunteers and men with erectile dysfunction not due to medical reasons. The stimuli from a receptive female and/or copulation itself lead to the release of dopamine (DA) in at least three integrative hubs. The nigrostriatal system promotes somatomotor activity; the mesolimbic system subserves numerous types of motivation and reward; and the medial preoptic nucleus (MPO) focuses the motivation onto specifically sexual targets, increases copulatory rate and efficiency, and coordinates genital reflexes. Accordingly, bupropion's lower rate of sexual dysfunction side effects may stem from its combined norepinephrine and dopamine reuptake inhibition. Orgasm releases dopamine in the nucleus accumbens in both men and women.

## D. Prolactin

Exton et al. (1999) investigated the cardiovascular, genital and endocrine changes in women after masturbation-induced orgasm. They reported orgasm-induced elevations of plasma epinephrine, norepinephrine and a long-lasting elevation of prolactin in addition to small increases in plasma LH and testosterone concentrations. In contrast, plasma concentrations of cortisol, FSH, beta-endorphin, progesterone, and estradiol were unaffected by orgasm. Prolactin released at orgasm might be responsible for the male refractory period necessary before developing a new erection. Dopamine agonists which serve as prolactin inhibiting agents, such as cabergoline, may reduce the refractory period in males (Kruger et al. 2003). This application is now utilized to treat anorgasmia or delayed orgasm by reducing the biological resistance to orgasm (Melmed, IsHak, and Berman 2005). More details are provided in Chapter 7 on Orgasmic Disorders.

### E. Oxytocin

Using a continuous blood sampling technique and anal electro-myography, Carmichael et al. (1994) reported a positive correlation between oxytocin levels and the intensity, but not duration, of orgasmic contractions in males and females. For multiorgasmic women, the amount of oxytocin level increase was positively correlated with subjective reports of orgasm intensity. Administration of oxytocin by nasal spray was reported to be effective in male anorgasmia in a recent case report (IsHak, Berman & Peters 2007). More details are provided in Chapter 7 on Orgasmic Disorders. Murphy et al. (1990) showed that naloxone inhibits oxytocin release at orgasm in men.

### F. Nitric Oxide

McCann et al. (2003) reviewed the role that NO plays at every level in the organism. In the brain, it activates the release of lutenizing hormone-releasing hormone (LHRH). The axons of the LHRH neurons project to the mating centers in the brain stem, and by efferent pathways, evoke the lordosis reflex in female rats. In normal males, the release of NO in the corpora cavernosa results in penile erection by generation of cyclic guanosine monophosphate (cGMP) that increases the blood flow into the penis. Phosophodiestrase–5 (PDE–5) catalyzes the degradation of cGMP. Sildenafil, vardenafil, and tadalafil all inhibit PDE–5, the end result is less degradation of cGMP which increases the amount of cGMP available to increase blood flow into the penis in response to sexual stimulation. NO also activates the release of LHRH, which reaches the pituitary and activates the release of gonadotropins by activating neural NO synthase (NOS) in the pituitary gland. Follicle stimulating hormone releasing hormone FSHRH selectively releases FSH also by activating NOS. Leptin releases LHRH by activating NOS to release FSH and LH with the same potency as LHRH. These actions are mediated by specific receptors on the gonadotropes for LHRH, FSHRH and Leptin. Gonadal steroids control the responsiveness of the pituitary. In the gonads, NO plays an important role inducing ovulation and in causing luteolysis; whereas in the reproductive tract, it relaxes uterine muscle via cGMP.

## G. Prostaglandins

Prostaglandins play a role in relaxing penile smooth musculature, which leads to more blood flow into the penis. Alprostadil is prostaglandin $E_1$ that facilitates erection by relaxation of trabecular smooth muscle and by dilation of cavernosal arteries. It be administered either as an intra-urethral suppository or directly injected into the corpora cavernosa. It has an immediate localized effect, which is synergistic when used with sildenafil.

## H. Sex Hormones

1. Testosterone:

In all mammals testosterone is critical for sexual behavior. Once a male is castrated he loses sexual activity. In rats this decline takes six to eight weeks. In man it takes one to two years. The slow decline may be for two reasons, one is the residual testosterone on receptors and the other is the prolonged response once the receptors are activated. If testosterone is supplemented exogenously at the time of castration, sexual activity is completely conserved. If it is supplemented later, sexual activity returns but it does so as gradually as it left. Neither the sites, nor mechanisms of action of testosterone have been completely elicited. Multiple sites of the brain are involved, but the preoptic area (POA) and anterior hypothalamus are two specific areas, which appear to stimulate copulatory behavior. The brain is involved by interacting with opioid and dopaminergic receptors in the ventral tegmental area (VTA) and ventral striatum. There, testosterone enhances recognition of cues sent by the female. There is a hypothesis that testosterone only affects sexual activity in males after being aromatized to estradiol. Its other metabolite dihydroxytestosterone may have a minor CNS effect or may simply support gonadal organs. Other reports show that dihydroxytestosterone can maintain copulatory behavior in man. In many species dihydroxytestosterone mediates sexual satiation, which is a state of sexual behavior inhibition that is attained after multiple ejaculations. Fernandez-Guasti et al. (2003) showed that androgen receptor immunoreactivity (AR) in the POA of sexually satiated rats was drastic when compared to that of animals ejaculating only once. These data reveal that sexual activity reduces AR activity in specific brain areas, and suggest the possibility that such a reduction underlies the sexual inhibition that characterizes sexual satiety. According to the Erectile Dysfunction Institute, after age forty, a man's testosterone level gradually declines. By age seventy, the level has normally decreased by about 30%. While this level is "normal" for a seventy year old man, it would be low for a younger man. Congenital disorders and anomalies (i.e. testicles) in the production of testosterone can specifically lead to the failed development of puberty and sexual desire in males. If such disorders have existed since birth, the lack of sexual desire and feeling should also have been absent since birth. Certain cancer treatments such as chemotherapy (as previously mentioned) and radiation therapy can directly damage the testicles, which can in turn lead to low sex drive amongst other complications. The use of high doses of estrogenic hormones in the treatment of prostate cancer will indeed cause a decrease in sexual desire. This treatment modality is aimed at reducing androgens (specifically testosterone). As a result, decreased libido along with erectile dysfunction can occur as early as two to four weeks following the initiation of treatment.

2. Estrogen

It has been established in animal models that estrogen restored sexual behavior in rats that had undergone oophorectomy. Estrogen increases the female rat's willingness to approach a male, and can enhance the production of stimuli that make her more attractive to the male (odors, pheromones, and vocalizations). Estrogen receptors, ER-alpha and ER-beta have been identified in numerous sites in the brain such as the arcuate nucleus, the POA, amygdala and the hippocampus. ER-alpha is present in the VMH nucleus and ER-beta in the paraventricular nucleus.

3. Progestins

It has been established in animal models that Progesterone facilitates the effects of estrogen on the sexual behavior in rats that had undergone oophorectomy. Progesterone has a biphasic effect.

First there is a transient rise in progesterone (following priming by estrogen), which stimulates sexually receptivity. Second, prolonged secretion of progesterone will inhibit sexual receptivity. This inhibitory effect is also associated with the role of progesterone in maintaining pregnancy.

## III. Pharmacological Agents and Sexual Dysfunction

A variety of substances (alcohol, illicit drugs, prescription and over the counter medications, dietary supplements, and toxins) exert negative effects on sexual functioning. This section will focus on some of the most commonly encountered substance in clinical practice.

### A. Overview of Medications Associated with Sexual Dysfunction

Among numerous classes of medications (Table 2), antihypertensives, psychotropic agents, and illicit drugs constitute some of the significant offenders.

Medications such as selective serotonin reuptake inhibitors and monoamine oxidase inhibitors used in the treatment of depression as well as benzodiazepines which are used in treating anxiety and antihypertensive medications can also impact desire and arousal. Medications with antihistaminic (i.e. benadryl) and anticholinergic (tricyclic antidepressants: elavil, benztropine) properties cause a decrease in vaginal lubrication (Sadock et al., 2003). Cigarette smoking by causing tissue damage through the release of free radicals has also been hypothesized in affecting vaginal lubrication and clitoral swelling.

The following medications could affect women's ability to achieve an orgasm and impede men's ability to ejaculate: selective serotonin reuptake inhibitors, narcotics, tricyclic antidepressants, methyldopa, amphetamines, antipsychotics, benzodiazepines, guanethedine, trazadone, and monoamine oxidase inhibitors.

### B. Sexual Dysfunction Associated with Antihypertensives

Both hypertension and anti-hypertensive drugs are associated with sexual dysfunction (Girerd 1996). A decrease in sexual desire was reported by 47% of men and 48% of women. Sexual arousal disturbance

**TABLE 1**

**Diagnostic Criteria for Substance-Induced Sexual Dysfunction**

A. Clinically significant sexual dysfunction that results in marked distress or interpersonal difficulty predominates in the clinical picture.

B. There is evidence from the history, physical examination, or laboratory findings that the sexual dysfunction is fully explained by substance use as manifested by either (1) or (2):

    (1) The symptoms in Criterion A developed during, or within a month of, Substance Intoxication

    (2) Medication use is etiologically related to the disturbance

C. The disturbance is not better accounted for by a Sexual Dysfunction that is not substance induced. Evidence that the symptoms are better accounted for by a Sexual Dysfunction that is not substance induced might include the following: the symptoms precede the onset of the substance use or Dependence (or medication use); the symptoms persist for a substantial period of time (e.g., about a month) after the cessation of intoxication, or are substantially in excess of what would be expected given the type or amount of the substance used or the duration of use; or there is other evidence that suggests the existence of an independent non-substance-induced Sexual Dysfunction (e.g., a history of recurrent non-substance-related episodes).

Note: This diagnosis should be made instead of a diagnosis of Substance Intoxication only when the sexual dysfunction is in excess of that usually associated with the intoxication syndrome and when the dysfunction is sufficiently severe to warrant independent clinical attention.

Code [Specific Substance]-Induced Sexual Dysfunction:

(291.8 (new code as of 10/01/96: 291.89) Alcohol; 292.89 Amphetamine [or Amphetamine-Like Substance]; 292.89 Cocaine; 292.89 Opioid; 292.89 Sedative, Hypnotic, or Anxiolytic; 292.89 Other [or Unknown] Substance)

Specify if:

    With Impaired Desire
    With Impaired Arousal
    With Impaired Orgasm
    With Sexual Pain

Specify if:

    With Onset During Intoxication: if the criteria are met for Intoxication with the substance and the symptoms develop during the intoxication syndrome

Reprinted with permission from the Diagnostic and Statistical Manual of Mental Disorders, Fourth Edition, Text Revision. Copyright 2000 American Psychiatric Association

---

**TABLE 2**

**Medications Associated with Sexual Dysfunction**

- Anticholesterol agents
- Antihypertensive agents
- Barbiturates
- Benzodiazepines
- Beta blockers
- Birth control pills
- Chemotherapeutic agents
- Clonidine
- Digoxin
- GnRH agonists
- H$_2$ blockers
- Indomethacin
- Ketoconazole
- Lithium
- Neuroleptics (antipsychotic agents)
- Oral contraceptives
- Phenytoin (Dilantin)
- Psychoactive agents
- Selective serotonin reuptake inhibitors
- Spirinolactone
- Tricyclic antidepressants

---

related to antihypertensive drugs occurs more often in men than in women. Both sexes may have difficulty achieving orgasm while taking antihypertensives. Eighty-two percent of women lack management of their sexual side effects, as do 54% of men. Modifications of antihypertensive treatments because of sexual side effects are rarely observed, on the order of 15% as reported by Girerd, 1996. Primary care physicians must consider sexual side effects when prescribing antihypertensive medication. There is evidence correlating diuretics, centrally acting sympatholytic drugs, and beta-blockers to higher incidences of sexual dysfunction. Calcium channel antagonists and angiotensin converting enzyme inhibitors cause less sexual dysfunction. (Fogari 2002). Other drugs used for the treatment of cardiac and cardiovascular diseases have been shown to negatively effect sexual function or even to cause or worsen sexual dysfunction.

In a community based epidemiological study of 1,709 men, analysis of data on multiple antihypertensive, vasodilator and cardiac medications revealed that digoxin use had the highest association with complete ED (Gupta 1998). The mechanism underlying digoxin-associated changes in sexual function remains poorly understood, but some scientists attributed sexual dysfunction to hormonal alterations observed with digoxin use; these changes include higher serum estrogen coupled with lower testosterone and luteinizing hormone levels. Some studies on human corpus cavernosum tissue indicate that sodium-pump activity also has a role in the regulation of erectile function, with pump inhibition causing contraction and diminution of NO induced relaxation. Gupta et al studied the effect of digoxin on sodium-pump activity in human corporeal smooth muscle strips in vitro and concluded that digoxin-associated alteration of human sexual function may be due to corporeal smooth muscle pump inhibition, which promotes contraction and impedes NO induced relaxation.

Beta blockers are believed to have negative effects on erectile function. Some theories point to adverse effects of decreased perfusion pressure, or a direct (but unknown) effect on smooth muscle. Beta-adrenergic blocking agents may cause ED by potentiating alpha–1 adreno-receptor-mediated contraction of corporal smooth muscle in the penis. It is unclear, however, why not all or even the majority of treated patients experience sexual dysfunction with beta-blocker use. A prospective, randomized, double-blind study showed that patients' sex lives were unaffected by metoprolol treatment (Franzen 2001), whiel other reported a higher incidence with propranolol and atenolol. Carvedilol has become a preferred agent for beta-blocker therapy in particular for patients with heart failure. A recent study comparing carvedilol with the angiotensin-receptor blocker valsartan demonstrated a decline in sexual activity within the carvedilol treated group. Notably, these patients were hypertensive treated with high doses of carvedilol, and patients with comorbidities such as diabetes mellitus and coronary atherosclerosis were excluded (Fogari 2001). Overall most beta-blockers appear to be associated with worsening of pre-existing erectile dysfunction in males It is not quite clear, however, whether beta-blockers do cause ED per se.

While sexual disorders caused by diuretics have been reported, the mechanism remains ill-defined. 10–20% of patients taking thiazide diuretics may experience a decline in sexual function. The aldosterone antagonist spironolactone is considered standard therapy for HF patients and also can cause erectile failure, gynecomastia, and decreased libido secondary to its anti-androgen effects. Many diuretics in fact also may cause decreased libido and impaired lubrication or impotence.

Croog et al found that the ACE-inhibitor captopril actually enhances sexual function (Croog 1986). It has been suggested that potential favorable sexual effects of captopril were secondary to improved cardiac function; however sufficient data to support this hypothesis do not exist. There is even less information available regarding the effects of ARBs on sexual function. Recent evidence suggests that losartan, an angiotensin II antagonist, is not associated with development of sexual dysfunction and might actually positively impact erectile function, sexual satisfaction, and frequency of sexual activity, as well as perceived quality of life, which recently also has been reported with candesartan and with valsartan (Fogari 2001, Schwarz 2006a).

Calcium Channel Blockers (CCBs) seem to cause fewer sexual problems than other antihypertensives; however, the same vasodilatation that causes decreased blood vessel constriction can also decrease the contractions essential for penile rigidity and orgasmic sensation. Other effects include decreasing dopamine activity, which increases prolactin, which can reduce sex drive, contribute to impotence, galactorrhea, and gynecomastia and block the actions of excitatory peptides that are involved in genital sensation, thus retarding ejaculation. CCBs can be used as a treatment to help reduce premature ejaculation. Few sexual effects from CCBs have been reported in women with normal sexual functioning. However, for women who already have sexual difficulties, side effects of CCBs that indirectly affect sexual function can include headache, flushing, swelling, bloating, dizziness, and weakness, which can dampen sexual desire and response. CCBs potentiate the effects of alcohol; therefore a few drinks combined with a CCB could possibly decrease sexual desire and function in both sexes.

The alpha-blocker, doxazosin, is another antihypertensive that may be beneficial for individuals with sexual dysfunction and hypertension. This alpha-blocker is a good choice for diabetic patients because it improves insulin sensitivity. Moreover, erectile dysfunction (ED) and hypertension are more prevalent among diabetics. Doxazosin and/or losartan can be beneficial in patients who develop ED after starting treatment with other antihypertensive drugs. These options could, in turn, ensure better compliance and blood pressure control. A fall in the overall cost of treatment can be anticipated if there is a reduced need for costly drugs prescribed for ED in patients with hypertension.

An effective way to treat hypertension and minimizes sexual dysfunction is by carefully choosing the anti-hypertensive agents. For example, diuretic can be combined with an ACE inhibitors or a Calcium Channel Blocker. However this is not often used in real practice (Khaja et al. 2003).

In patients receiving antihypertensive drugs or any cardiovascular medication concomitant use of some oral agents for ED, which have vasodilator properties, may result in a reduction in blood pressure. This is, generally, mild and not likely to be of clinical concern. No statistically significant differences were observed by Kloner et al. (1992). They found that administration of a potent, selective, reversible phosphodiesterase–5 inhibitor is safe in patients receiving a concomitant antihypertensive agent. The concomitant use of any available PDE–5 inhibitor (sildenafil, vardenafil, tadalafil) and organic nitrates or NO donators, whether it is in oral, sublingual, intravenous or any other form is, however, absolutely contraindicated within several half-lives of either drug because it may lead to a potentiation of the decreases in blood pressure and thus cause life-threatening hypotension. In patients receiving medication for any cardiovascular condition which worsens sexual function or causes even dysfunction, however, careful evaluation of potential drug side effects and if possible—exchange of medication to classes without sexual side effects is encouraged, but unfortunately not frequently done since the health care providers often might not be aware of the patients' problem (Schwarz 2006b).

## C. Psychotropic Medications

It is common to experience sexual dysfunction with the use of many psychiatric medications, but it is important to understand that the psychiatric illness being treated may be the cause of the sexual difficulties. Controlled studies have shown that 70% to 80% of depressed patients have diminished libido. Anorgasmia is one helpful symptom in distinguishing between depression-related and treatment-related sexual difficulties. Anorgasmia is rarely due to depression alone.

1. SSRIs can cause problems in any phase of the sexual response cycle. Most common complaints are of delayed orgasm, complete lack of orgasm, or ejaculatory difficulties. The effects of SSRIs on sexual

**TABLE 3**

**Incidence of SSRI-induced Sexual Side Effects in Women (Kanaly & Berman 2002)**

| Medication | Incidence (%) |
|------------|---------------|
| fluoxetine | 57.7 |
| sertraline | 62.9 |
| fluvoxamone | 62.3 |
| paroxetine | 70.7 |
| citalopram | 72.7 |
| venlafaxine | 67.3 |
| mirtazapine | 24.4 |
| nefazodone | 8.0 |
| amineptine | 6.9 |
| moclobemide | 3.9 |

functioning seem strongly dose-related and can vary among the individual SSRI depending on the extent of the serotonin and dopamine reuptake mechanisms, anticholinergic effects, and accumulation over time.

Sexual side effects of SSRIs should not be viewed as entirely negative; some studies have shown improved control of premature ejaculation in men.

A variety of strategies have been reported in the management of SSRI-induced sexual dysfunction:

a. One option is to observe the patient until after the first six weeks of SSRI therapy, the sexual side effects may resolve in some cases. Sexual dysfunction secondary to depression tends to improve with treatment.

b. Decreasing the dosage may eliminate the sexual dysfunction. SSRIs have a flat dose-response curve, meaning that there may be flexibility to lower the dosage enough to eliminate the side effect while maintaining therapeutic efficacy. Pay close attention to signs of recurrent depression and increase the dose again if necessary.

c. Adding a PDE–5 inhibitor has been proven to be one of the most effective strategies for both men and women. Dosing and side effects are detailed in Chapter 4 on Biopsychosocial Evaluation and Treatment of Sexual Disorders.

d. Adding (or cross tapering to) bupropion and its sustained-release form (Wellbutrin-SR) at 300 mg per day had been shown to improve sexual function in placebo-controlled trials (Ashton et al. 1998 and Clayton et al. 2004).

e. Adding buspirone (Buspar), a non-benzodiazepine anxiolytic, was found to be effective at 20–30 mg bid in a retrospective study of 16 patients by Norden (1994). Eleven of the 16 patients returned to near normal functioning; the rest had less than 50% improvement. The drug caused increased irritability in some patients. A retrospective analysis of data from a placebo-controlled trial showed that of 47 patients experiencing SSRI-induced sexual dysfunction, 58% reported improvement within the first week of daily buspirone treatment, whereas 25% to 30% of patients taking placebo reported better sexual functioning.

f. Cross tapering to mirtazapine (Remeron) at 15–45 mg per day.

g. Adding cyproheptadine (Periactin) at 8 mg per day, which is an antihistaminic with antiserotonergic properties, may exert its beneficial effect because it antagonizes the $5\text{-HT}_{2A}$ receptor.

h. Yohimbine at 5.4 mg, 2–3 times per day may be effective in treating sexual dysfunction. A retrospective case review of 45 patients by Ashton et al (1997) compared yohimbine, cyproheptadine, and amantadine as treatments for SSRI-induced sexual dysfunction. Of the 21 patients taking yohimbine, 17 (81%) showed improvement in sexual functioning while only 48% of those taking cyproheptadine and 42% of those taking amantadine did so. The treatments had a low rate of adverse effects. Agitation occurred in three patients taking yohimbine, sedation and weight gain in two patients taking cyproheptadine, and depressive symptoms developed in one patient taking amantadine.

i. Adding ephedrine at 50 mg one hour prior to sexual intercourse for women on SSRIs had shown increased sexual performance but placebo produced almost similar effects (Meston 2004).

However, the FDA believes that ephedrine (in ephedra) may be related to more than 50 deaths. Most of the serious injuries involve high blood pressure that can cause bleeding in the brain, a stroke or a heart attack. In February 2004, The FDA issued a regulation prohibiting the sale of dietary supplements containing ephedrine alkaloids.

j. Reboxetine is a Noradrenaline reuptake inhibitor antidepressant has proven in multicenter, randomized, 8-week, double blind study of 450 patients to have sexual side effects similar to placebo. This medication is not FDA approved in the US (Clayton et al. 2003).

## 2. Antipsychotics

Sexual dysfunction is frequent in treatment of schizophrenia, especially in men. It may be a direct consequence of dopamine antagonism, combined with indirect effects of increased prolactin. Atypical antipsychotics are associated with a lower incidence of adverse sexual events than conventional antipsychotics. For example, there is a dose-related increase in prolactin with risperidone whereas olanzapine is associated with mild and transient increases in prolactin during long-term treatment. Treatment with clozapine does not result in prolactin elevation, but the risk of agranulocytosis restricts its use to frequent laboratory monitoring. Olanzapine, and ziprasidone cause transient increases in prolactin. Quetiapine has no more effect on serum prolactin than placebo. Together with its low frequency of reproductive or hormonal side effects and a low incidence of extrapyramidal symptoms, the tolerability profile of quetiapine may be particularly beneficial for many patients. Sexual dysfunction can be an important source of distress to patients and adversely affects compliance, and is one of the factors that must be taken into account when selecting treatment (Cutler 2003).

## D. Alcohol, Illicit Drugs, and Nicotine

### 1. Ethanol

Shakespeare once said of alcohol as "lechery...it provokes and unprovokes; it provokes the desire but it takes away the performance." Alcohol can decrease inhibitions and increase the likelihood of engaging in sex but less capable of the act.

In small amounts, alcohol can reduce inhibitions and increase sexual desire in both sexes. Although small amounts of alcohol may increase sexual desire, it does not necessarily increase sexual arousal. Even in small doses ethanol causes men's erections to be less firm.

In larger doses alcohol reduces sexual arousal in both sexes. In men, alcohol causes impotence through several mechanisms. Long-term use of alcohol reduces testosterone levels and increases estrogen levels, which can result in impotence. Short-term use can cause transient impotence through alcohol's sedative effect. Additionally, alcohol can affect the nerves of the penis, causing neurogenic impotence.

Alcohol also reduces sexual arousal in women. Alcohol can reduce vaginal lubrication by causing the body to send less blood to the genital region. In moderate or large quantities, alcohol can make orgasm difficult to achieve for women, just as it can for men.

Hormonal changes caused by long-term alcohol use can cause a reduction in libido, in addition to causing impotence. Using alcohol in combination with other depressants can amplify this effect.

Alcohol can interfere with the production of sperm in men by producing abnormalities in sperm, making them less motile. When alcohol-effected sperm causes a pregnancy, there is a greater likelihood of miscarriage or birth defects.

Some agree that sex is less enjoyable when under the influence of alcohol; because alcohol makes the penis less sensitive and because it takes men take longer to reach orgasm. Men are also often less interested in pleasing their partner when intoxicated.

## 2. Marijuana

For the first half-hour after consuming marijuana, the drug causes excitement and euphoria and increases the user's heart rate. The user may interpret these effects as sexual excitement. However, after half an hour, marijuana has a sedative effect.

Long-term use of marijuana generally has a negative effect on sexuality. Chronic heavy use of marijuana can lower the libido. There is some evidence that it can cause erectile dysfunction as well. In women, marijuana can disrupt the menstrual cycle in long-term use.

Long-term use of marijuana can lower sperm production or cause sperm to develop abnormally. It can also lower testosterone levels. Both of these effects go away after marijuana use ceases.

Many people find sex under the influence of marijuana to be especially enjoyable. According to "Adverse Drug Effects" by Jennifer Kelly, marijuana "enhances sensory experiences, and so is described by some as an aphrodisiac." Some feel that marijuana makes orgasms longer and more intense. This may be a result of the distorted sense of time that marijuana intoxication causes. Studies have found no measurable differences in the length or intensity of the orgasms of people under the influence of marijuana, even when the subjects felt that their orgasms had been longer and more intense.

Marijuana does not always make sex more enjoyable. In people who are unfamiliar with the drug or are in unfamiliar situations, Marijuana sometimes causes anxiety and self-consciousness. These emotions can interfere with sexual desire. Motor skills are also impaired by marijuana making the user clumsy, which can reduce one's performance during sex.

### 3. Cocaine

As with all of the stimulants, cocaine can cause erectile dysfunction but in moderate doses, the effect of neurogenic contraction of penile trabecular smooth muscle may lead to priapism. Men generally find it very difficult to ejaculate on high doses of cocaine, which some see as an advantage, and some find it frustrating. Finally, in very high doses, cocaine can cause spontaneous orgasm, but doses this high can be fatal.

In small doses, cocaine causes excitement and euphoria, which the user may interpret as sexual excitement. Chronic heavy use of cocaine can lower the libido. Due to the cocaine's addictive nature, the desire for cocaine may eventually overpower any desire for sex.

Cocaine is a local anesthetic. When applied to the skin, it reduces sensitivity. Some men take advantage of this effect by rubbing the drug on their penises so as to delay orgasm; however this reduces sensation. The same effect can be achieved legally and relatively inexpensively through anesthetizing creams.

Ephedrine and cocaine: Anecdotal evidence suggests that priapism may result from ephedrine use. The effects of cocaine and ephedrine on adrenergic regulation of cavernosal tissue and the potential role of sympathetic dysregulation in the development of priapism have not been studied. One study by Munarriz tested rabbit penile cavernosal tissue strips in organ bath preparations were subjected to electrical field stimulation (EFS) in the absence or presence of ephedrine or cocaine. Ephedrine and cocaine initially caused contractions in cavernosal tissue strips that persisted for several hours. EFS-induced contractions became attenuated over time in tissues treated with ephedrine or cocaine. Eventually, the contractile responses to EFS were not distinguishable from the basal tone, although the tissues remained responsive to exogenous phenylephrine. Functional activation of alpha-adrenergic receptors on trabecular smooth muscle does not appear to be impaired with prolonged cocaine or ephedrine exposure. However, chronic use of cocaine or ephedrine may deplete norepinephrine from sympathetic nerve terminals, leading to priapism (Munarriz 2003).

### 4. Amphetamine and stimulants

Like alcohol, amphetamine like drugs, including methamphetamine and MDMA (ecstasy), "provoke the desire but take away the performance." Amphetamine like drugs can increase one's desire for sex. In men, amphetamine often makes achieving and maintaining an erection difficult. Conversely, in moderate doses, amphetamine may occasionally cause priapism, Male amphetamine users report penile shrinkage. Because of the erection difficulties and penile shrinkage amphetamine like drugs cause, men on amphetamines often find masturbation easier than sex.

In spite of the erection difficulties amphetamines cause, male amphetamine users find it possible, although difficult, to achieve orgasm while flaccid when they are on amphetamines. Men generally find it very difficult to ejaculate while on high doses of amphetamines. Some people see this as an advantage, because it allows men to last longer during sex. However, this side effect can also be very frustrating. They feel that the physical sensation of sexual stimulation is better while on amphetamines, but the overall experience is less enjoyable.

Ejaculation can cause mild discomfort to men on amphetamines. Male amphetamine users report that ejaculation feels equally good and satisfying whether on or off amphetamines, however they report testicular discomfort after ejaculating while on amphetamines. In very high doses, amphetamines can also cause spontaneous orgasm. However, doses this high are extremely dangerous, as they can cause convulsions, heart failure, stroke and death.

## 5. Opioids

Opioids can reduce sexual responses in both sexes. Men on opiates have difficulty achieving erections and ejaculating, while women on heroin produce less vaginal lubrication and have more difficulty reaching orgasm. Heavy use of opiates can lower the libido.

## 6. Amyl Nitrate and Butyl Nitrate (poppers)

Poppers are often used as sexual enhancers. They release nitric oxide causing erection and relaxation of the rectum facilitating anal sex. They cause a feeling of heat and excitement which some feel makes sex more enjoyable. Although they can be legally purchased, poppers can increase the risk of heart failure.

## 7. GHB

In small doses, the effects of GHB are similar to those of alcohol. At low doses, GHB decreases inhibitions and increases sexual desire. However, the potency of this drug is often unpredictable, and in doses only slightly larger dose than are taken recreationally, it can cause the user to vomit or pass out and can even result in death. GHB is particularly dangerous in combination with ethanol and other depressants. It is reported to be used as a tool for date rape since it is clear, odorless, and almost tasteless, not easily detected, and because of its sedative effect.

## 8. Nicotine

Nicotine can affect erectile tissue and the muscles involved in producing an erection, thus causing impotence. Men who smoke tobacco are twice as likely to be impotent as non-smoking men of the same age. Using nicotine in combination with cardiac drugs, antihypertensive medications or vasodilators drastically increase the probability of complete impotence.

Nicotine can cause men to produce fewer sperm, and can cause deformities in the remaining sperm. These deformities reduce the motility of the sperm, and in pregnancies caused by these deformed sperm there is a greater chance of miscarriage or health problems for the fetus.

## IV. Conclusion

Substance induced sexual dysfunction is a common phenomenon. It can be either a side effect of a substance or a direct effect of a substance. There has been a lot of exciting discoveries of new medications that enable physicians to treat multiple diseases in new ways. These new medications have helped us gain a better understanding of how the sexual function can be affected with different neurotransmitters, hormone, or the substance itself through the sexual dysfunction in treated patients. Sometimes the physician is faced with the dilemma of making decision between medication benefits versus side effects. It is important to obtain informed consent and ask for any changes in the sexual functioning through out the course of treatment. The involvement of the patient in the decision making process will help to reduce dissatisfaction and to increase the awareness of sexual dysfunction. The temporal course of developing sexual dysfunction along with medication changes can be an important clue to the cause of sexual dysfunction. Normal healthy sex is very much a part of human life and the effects of any medication or substance need to be considered and treated for the better quality of life in patients.

## *References*

Argiolas A, Melis MR: The neurophysiology of the sexual cycle. Journal of Endocrinological Investigation 26(3 Suppl):20–2, 2003

Ashton AK, Hamer R, Rosen RC: Serotonin reuptake inhibitor-induced sexual dysfunction and its treatment: A large-scale retrospective study of 596 psychiatric outpatients. J Sex Marital Ther 23:165, 1997

Ashton AK, Rosen RC: Bupropion as an antidote for serotonin reuptake inhibitor-induced sexual function. J Clin Psychiatry 59:112, 1998

Bancroft J: Sexual desire and the brain. Sexual & Marital Therapy Vol 3(1) 11–27, 1988

Bancroft J: The medicalization of female sexual dysfunction: the need for caution. Archives of Sexual Behavior 31(5):451–5, 2002

Beauregard M, Levesque J, Bourgouin P: Neural correlates of conscious self-regulation of emotion. Journal of Neuroscience 21(18):RC165, 2001

Carmichael MS, Warburton VL, Dixen J, Davidson JM. Relationships among cardiovascular, muscular, and oxytocin responses during human sexual activity. Arch Sex Behav. 1994;23:59–77

Clayton AH, Warnock JK, Kornstein SG, et al: A placebo-controlled trial of bupropion SR as an antidote for selective serotonin reuptake inhibitor-induced sexual dysfunction: J Clin Psychiatry 65(1):62–7, 2004

Clayton AH, Zajecka J, Ferguson JM, et al.: Lack of sexual dysfunction with the selective noradrenaline reuptake inhibitor reboxetine during treatment for major depressive disorder. Int Clin Psychopharmacol. 18(3):151–6, 2003

Cohn BA: In search of human skin pheromones. Arch Dermatol. 130: 1048–1051, 1994

Croog SH, Levine S, Testa MA, Brown B, Bulpitt CJ, Jenkins CD, Klerman GL, Williams GH. The effects on antihypertensive therapy on quality of life. New Engl J Med 1986; 314:1657–1664.

Cutler AJ: Sexual dysfunction and antipsychotic treatment. Psychoneuroendocri nology. 28 Suppl 1:69–82, 2003

Exton MS. Bindert A. Kruger T. Scheller F. Hartmann U. Schedlowski M. Cardiovascular and endocrine alterations after masturbation-induced orgasm in women.[see comment]. Psychosomatic Medicine 61(3):280–9, 1999

Fernandez-Guasti, Alonso; Swaab, Dick; Rodriguez-Manzo, Gabriela. Sexual behavior reduces hypothalamic androgen receptor immunoreactivity. Psychoneuroendocrinology 28(4) 501–512, 2003

Fogari R, Zoppi A, Poletti L, Marasi G, Mugellini A, and Corradi L. Sexual activity in hypertensive men treated with valsartan or carvedilol: a crossover study. Am J Hypertens 2001; 14:27–31.

Franzen D, Metha A, Seifert N, Braun M, Hopp HW. Effects of beta-blockers on sexual performance in men with coronary heart disease. A prospective randomized and double blinded study. Intl J Impotence Res 2001; 13:348–351.

Goldhill J: Male and female sexual dysfunction: Blockbuster indication for multiple pharmacological targets. Lead Discovery Ltd, http://www.leaddiscovery.co.uk/target-discovery/abstracts/dossier-MDI002.html, 2002

Gupta S, Salimpour P, Saenz de Tejada I, Daley J, Gholami S, Daller M, Krane RJ, Traish AM, Goldstein I. A possible mechanism for alteration of human erectile function by digoxin: Inhibition of corpus cavernosum sodium/potassium adenosine triphosphate activity. J Urol 1998; 159:1529–1536.

Hatfield, Elaine; Rapson, Richard L. Passionate love and sexual desire: Cultural and historical perspectives. Vangelisti, Anita L. (Ed); Reis, Harry T. (Ed); et al. Stability and change in relationships. Advances in personal relationships. New York, NY, Cambridge University Press, 2002, pp 306–324

Heaton JP, Adams MA: Update on central function relevant to sex: remodeling the basis of drug treatments for sex and the brain. International Journal of Impotence Research 15 Suppl 5:S25–32, 2003

Hofman MA, Swaab DF: Sexual dimorphism of the human brain: myth and reality. Experimental & Clinical Endocrinology 98(2):161–70, 1991

Holstege G. Georgiadis JR. The emotional brain: neural correlates of cat sexual behavior and human male ejaculation. Progress in Brain Research 143:39–45, 2004

Hsieh GC, Hollingsworth PR, Martino B, et al.: Central mechanisms regulating penile erection in conscious rats: the dopaminergic systems related to the proerectile effect of apomorphine. Journal of Pharmacology & Experimental Therapeutics 308(1):330–8, 2004

Hull EM, Lorrain DS, Du J, Matuszewich L,Lumley LA, Putnam SK, Moses J Hormone-neurotransmitter interactions in the control of sexual behavior 14260–4110, USA Behav Brain Res 105(1):105–16, 1999

IsHak, WW, Berman D, Peters A: Male Anorgasmia Trreated with Oxytocin. The Journal of Sexual Medicine (in press)

Kanaly KA and Berman JR: Sexual Side Effects of SSRI Medications: Potential Treatment Strategies for SSRI-induced Female Sexual Dysfunction. Current Women's Health Reports 2:409–416, 2002

Kaplan HS: Disorders of Sexual Desire. New York, NY, Brunner/Mazel Inc, 1979

Karama S, Lecours AR, Leroux JM, et al.: Areas of brain activation in males and females during viewing of erotic film excerpts. Human Brain Mapping 16(1):1–13, 2002

Kruger TH, Haake P, Haverkamp J, Kramer M, Exton MS, Saller B, Leygraf N, Hartmann U, and Schedlowski M: Effects of acute prolactin manipulation on sexual drive and function in males. Journal of Endocrinology 179(3):357–365, 2003

Levin RJ: The mechanisms of human female sexual arousal. Annu Rev Sex Res. 3:1–48, 1992

Masters WH, Johnson VE: Human Sexual Response. Boston, Mass, Little Brown & Co Inc, 1966

McCann SM, Haens G, Mastronardi C, et al.: The role of nitric oxide (NO) in control of LHRH release that mediates gonadotropin release and sexual behavior. Current Pharmaceutical Design 9(5):381–90, 2003

McKenna KE: Neural circuitry involved in sexual function. Journal of Spinal Cord Medicine 24(3):148–54, 2001

McKenna KE: The neurophysiology of female sexual function. World Journal of Urology 20(2):93–100, 2002

Melmed S, IsHak WW, Berman D: Use Of Cabergoline For The Treatment of Anorgasmia or Delayed Orgasm, in IsHak WW: Orgasmic Disorders, Sexual Medicine Course. Presented at the American Psychiatric Association annual meeting in Atlanta, GA, May 2005

Meston CM, Frohlich PF: The Neurobiology of Sexual Function. Arch Gen Psychiatry 57:1012–1030, 2000

Meston CM: A randomized, placebo-controlled, crossover study of ephedrine for SSRI-induced female sexual dysfunction. J Sex Marital Ther. 30(2):57–68, 2004

Millan MJ. Peglion JL. Lavielle G. Perrin-Monneyron S: 5-HT2c receptors mediate penile erections in rats: actions of novel and selective agonists and antagonists. European Journal of Pharmacology 325(1):9–12, 1997

Munarriz R. Hwang J. Goldstein I, et al.: Cocaine and ephedrine-induced priapism: case reports and investigation of potential adrenergic mechanisms. Urology 62(1):187–92, 2003

Norden MJ: Buspirone treatment of sexual dysfunction associated with selective serotonin reuptake inhibitors. Depression 2:109, 1994

Pfaus JG: Neurobiology of sexual behavior. Current Opinion in Neurobiology 9(6)751–758, 1999

Porges SW: Love: an emergent property of the mammalian autonomic nervous system. Psychoneuroendocrinology 23(8):837–61, 1998

Rajfer, J, Aronson, WJ, Bush, PA, Dorey, FJ and Ignarro, LJ: Nitric oxide as a mediator of relaxation of the corpus cavernosum in response to nonadrenergic, noncholinergic neurotransmission. N. Engl. J. Med. 326: 90–94, 1992

Rampin O: Pharmacology of alpha-adrenoceptors in male sexual function. European Urology 36 Suppl 1:103–6, 1999

Schwarz ER (a), Rasatogi S, Kapur V, Sulemanjee N, Rodriguez JJ. Erectile dysfunction in heart failure patients. J Am Coll Cardiol, in press, 2006

Schwarz ER (b). Sex and the Heart, Friedel & Ernst Academic Press, Los Angeles, 2006

# 4

# Sexual Dysfunction Due to General Medical Conditions

WAGUIH WILLIAM ISHAK, M.D.
ROD AMIRI, M.D.
ERNST R. SCHWARZ, M.D., PH.D.

## I. Introduction

According to the DSM-IV-TR (APA 2000), sexual dysfunction is diagnosed when the problem has caused marked distress or interpersonal difficulty. Sexual dysfunction can be the result of psychological and physiological factors or a combination of the two. The objective of this chapter is to introduce sexual dysfunctions that are due to a general medical condition. In order to conclude that a physiologic factor or medical condition is responsible for a sexual dysfunction, it is necessary that the history, physical examination, and laboratory findings provide the evidence that the general medical condition is directly responsible for the occurrence of the specific dysfunction.

## TABLE 1
## Diagnostic Criteria for Sexual Dysfunction Due to . . .
## [Indicate the General Medical Condition]

A. Clinically significant sexual dysfunction that results in marked distress or interpersonal difficulty predominates in the clinical picture.

B. There is evidence from the history, physical examination, or laboratory findings that the sexual dysfunction is fully explained by the direct physiological effects of a general medical condition.

C. The disturbance is not better accounted for by another mental disorder (e.g., Major Depressive Disorder).

Select code and term based on the predominant sexual dysfunction:

625.8 Female Hypoactive Sexual Desire Disorder Due to . . . [Indicate the General Medical Condition]: if deficient or absent sexual desire is the predominant feature

608.89 Male Hypoactive Sexual Desire Disorder Due to . . . [Indicate the General Medical Condition]: if deficient or absent sexual desire is the predominant feature

607.84 Male Erectile Disorder Due to . . . [Indicate the General Medical Condition]: if male erectile dysfunction is the predominant feature

625.0 Female Dyspareunia Due to . . . [Indicate the General Medical Condition]: if pain associated with intercourse is the predominant feature

608.89 Male Dyspareunia Due to . . . [Indicate the General Medical Condition]: if pain associated with intercourse is the predominant feature

625.8 Other Female Sexual Dysfunction Due to . . . [Indicate the General Medical Condition]: if some other feature is predominant (e.g., Orgasmic Disorder) or no feature predominates

608.89 Other Male Sexual Dysfunction Due to . . . [Indicate the General Medical Condition]: if some other feature is predominant (e.g., Orgasmic Disorder) or no feature predominates

Coding note: Include the name of the general medical condition on Axis I, e.g., 607.84 Male Erectile Disorder Due to Diabetes Mellitus; also code the general medical condition on Axis III.

Reprinted with permission from the Diagnostic and Statistical Manual of Mental Disorders, Fourth Edition, Text Revision. Copyright 2000 American Psychiatric Association

Sexual dysfunctions due to medical conditions include: disorders of desire, arousal, orgasm, and sexual pain disorders. The information provided would focus on the most common medical and physiologic conditions, which can potentially lead to any of the four distinct types of sexual disorders (Golombok et al 1984). The existing treatments will be highlighted.

## II. Medical Conditions Affecting Sexual Functioning

A.  Autoimmune: systemic lupus erythematosus

B.  Cardiovascular: coronary artery disease, heart failure, cardiac arrhythmia, cerebrovascular disease, hypertension, generalized atherosclerosis and peripheral vascular disease, anemia

C.  Congenital: deformities, genital abnormalities

D.  Endocrinal/hormonal: hyperthyroidism, hypothyroidism, diabetes mellitus, hyperprolactinemia, low testosterone, low estrogen

E.  Genetic: Turner's syndrome, Androgen Insensitivity Syndrome, Klinefelter Syndrome, Down Syndrome

F.  Infectious: HIV, encephalitis, meningitis, pelvic inflammatory disease, syphilis, UTI

G.  Metabolic: vitamin deficiencies, hypercholesterolemia, morbid obesity

H.  Musculoskeletal: fibromyalgia, arthritis, back problems resulting in pain.

I.  Neoplastic: pelvic tumors, brain tumors, pituitary tumors

J.  Neurological: parkinson's disease, peripheral neuropathy, multiple sclerosis

K.  Pelvic/genito-urinary: endometriosis, prostatic hypertrophy, incontinence, pelvic organ prolapse, Peyronie's disease

L.  Traumatic: pelvic injuries and surgery, head injury

Other conditions that can affect sexual function are advanced age, chronic diseases in general, malnutrition as well as medication side effects, nicotine, drug and alcohol use and abuse.

## III.  Desire Disorders Due to General Medical Conditions

Hypoactive sexual desire disorder is characterized by persistent or recur-rently deficient (or absent) sexual fantasies and desire for sexual activity. The judgment of deficiency or absence is typically made by the clinician who takes into account factors such as age or context of the individual's life. Aging, some of the above described medical conditions, and surgical procedures can affect sexual desire.

A.  Chronic illnesses that deplete the individual's energy or compel the person to adapt and make life long adjustments can lead to depression and anxiety, which in turn affect sex, drive.

B.  Surgical/gynecological interventions such as a hysterectomy, ileostomy and mastectomy can significantly affect body image, and make women feel less feminine and sexual. Additionally, decreased blood flow to the pelvic region following surgery involving the pelvic floor, abdomen, bladder, and genitals or due to a medical condition such as diabetes or atherosclerosis can directly and indirectly impair sexual desire.

C.  Even though the relationship between sexual desire and sex hormones is not fully understood, both men and women experience sexual desire difficulties with altered hormonal levels.

    1.  Decreased sex drive and absence of sexual fantasies were observed to be the result of decreased estrogen. Hormone replacement therapy can restore hormone levels affected by age, hormone dysfunction, or surgery to normal levels thereby restoring sexual desire and func-tion (Bachmann & Leiblum 2004). Estrogen's effect on sex drive is thought to be indirect, by enhancing mood, vasomotor symptoms, and genital atrophy.

    2.  Conversely, studies involving progesterone (another female hormone) demonstrated that it might have a negative impact on sexual desire by affecting mood and the availability of androgens (sex hormones).

    3.  Androgens are thought to influence sexual function in both males and females by their effects on sexual motivation and desire; low

testosterone levels as well have been correlated with sexual infrequency and reduced libido. Braunstein et al. (2005) tested a testosterone transdermal patch showing its effectiveness in the treatment of sexual desire disorder in surgically menopausal women.

4. An excess of prolactin, a hormone which in adults regulates the behavioral aspects of reproduction and infant care (Sadock 2004), can lead to diminished libido in both males and females. Treatment of the underlying cause of hyperprolactinemia (high blood prolactin levels) with medication or through surgical intervention (i.e. removal of a pituitary gland tumor) has been shown to restore sexual drive. Anti-prolactin dopamine agonists such as bromocriptine and cabergoline had shown effectiveness in restoring sexual functioning though the normalization of prolactin levels.

## IV. Arousal Disorders Due to General Medical Conditions

Sexual arousal disorders are categorized by the DSM-IV-TR into female and male sexual arousal disorders. According to Sadock et al., this diagnosis considers the focus, intensity, and duration of sexual activity in which individuals engage. If sexual stimulation is inadequate in focus, intensity, or duration, the diagnosis should not be made. Female Sexual Arousal Disorder occurs when the female has insufficient vaginal lubrication and clitoral swelling. A man is considered to have arousal difficulties when he is unable to attain or maintain an adequate erection, which leads to erectile dysfunction.

A. **Female Sexual Arousal Disorder** may be caused by various psychological and physical conditions. The process of clitoral swelling and vaginal lubrication directly rely upon the adequate flow of blood to the vaginal area. Any medical condition which hampers this process can affect the ability of a woman to become aroused during sexual activity (Basson 2002). To make a diagnosis of an underlying medical cause, the physician must take a thorough medical and sexual history, conduct a physical examination with review of the organ systems, and evaluate laboratory examinations in order to determine that a general medical condition is responsible for the sexual arousal disorder. Physiologic diagnostic tests can be useful in aiding the physician to measure vaginal blood flow and engorgement. Through vaginal photoplethysmography, an acrylic tampon-shaped instrument is inserted in the vagina in order to measure blood flow and temperature. Vaginal pH testing utilizes a probe to detect bacteria which lead to vaginal tissue inflammation. The normally acidic pH of the vagina is protective against disease causing pathogens. Diminished vaginal secretions and hormone levels commonly seen in peri- and postmenopausal women can make the vaginal pH more basic which is then readily detected with this instrument. A biothesiometer is an instrument, which can examine the sensitivity of the labia and clitoris to pressure and temperature.

1. Pelvic problems such as endometriosis (the presence of uterine tissue outside of the uterus), cystitis (bladder infection), or vaginitis (inflammation of vaginal tissue which leads to vaginal dryness and decreased arousal) can all lead to arousal disorder. Treating the underlying cause responsible for the arousal disorder through surgical intervention (i.e. endometriosis), or the use of antibiotics for the treatment of urinary tract infections can alleviate symptoms of arousal disorder.

2. Endocrine (hormone) problems such as diabetes, which leads to nerve end damage, hormone changes, and decreased blood flow, and hypothyroidism, can also lead to sexual arousal disorder. With some diabetic patients, diligent blood sugar control has shown to be effective in alleviating symptoms of poor clitoral swelling and vaginal lubrication. Additionally, normalizing thyroid hormone levels may be helpful in restoring arousal in hypothyroid female patients.

3. High blood pressure and heart disease are also systemic conditions which have been implicated in diminishing sexual arousal. Sexual frigidity and dissatisfaction leading to sexual dysfunction, at least for a prolonged period of time has been reported in women after myocardial infarction (Abramov 1976, Vacanti 2005).

4. Surgical procedures such as hysterectomy or mastectomy can affect a woman's sense of femininity and in turn affect sexual desire and arousal.

5. Hormonal fluctuations and changes that accompany natural female processes such as pregnancy and menopause may indeed diminish sexual arousal.

B.  **Male Erectile Disorder (ED)** may be also caused by psychological, physiological (due to a medical condition or drugs), or a combination of both. Any condition which affects the man having an adequate blood pressure to carry blood to the penis, or causes any "leaks" in the penile venous system can lead to erectile dysfunction. Additionally, a male must have adequate levels of testosterone in order to have an erection. As with other sexual dysfunctions, a thorough medical/sexual history, physical examination, and laboratory examinations must be conducted by the physician in order to determine that a physical cause is responsible for erectile dysfunction. The physical examination should focus on secondary sexual characteristics, an abdominal examination, pulse examination, S2-S4 neurological assessment, and external genitalia examination. An abdominal examination could reveal an abdominal aortic aneurysm, which statistics have shown to be responsible for about one percent of all cases of erectile dysfunction. The major lower extremity pulses, specifically the femoral and popliteal pulses are important markers for systemic atherosclerotic disease. An assessment of S2-S4 neural pathways can rule out a diagnosis of neurogenic erectile dysfunction. Laboratory evaluation should include hematological and metabolic laboratory analyses as recommended by the National Institute of Health (NIH) consensus panel. The screen should also include a measure of serum glucose in order to rule out diabetes. Assessment of thyroid and liver function tests can also offer value in ruling out any abnormalities in these organs. Hormonal assessment is also paramount, and total and free testosterone levels along with LH and prolactin levels should be measured.

A number of tests and investigations may be helpful in aiding the physician to determine a cause for a male's erectile dysfunction. These tests include: vascular testing such as duplex ultrasound and dynamic infusion cavernosometry, nocturnal penile tumescence and rigidity analysis, and somatosensory evoked potentials and pudendal electromyelography. Though controversial, these tests are chiefly reserved for patients who have a high chance of being cured such as patients with psychogenic ED, young males with arteriogenic ED secondary to trauma, and males with crural leaks.

Compiled data from the Bureau of Health Statistics, the National Cancer Institute, the American Diabetes Association, and the American Cancer Society have revealed that of all of the cases of erectile dysfunction caused by physical factors, forty percent is due to vascular disease, thirty percent is a result of diabetes, eleven percent is secondary to medications, drug abuse, and hormone deficiency, ten percent is a result of neurological disorders, and nine percent of all physical cases of ED is due to pelvic surgery and trauma.

These numbers declare that the majority of cases of male erectile dysfunction, therefore, has a vasculogenic origin, namely is caused by a condition called "endothelial dysfunction".

## 1. Endothelial dysfunction

Endothelial dysfunction has gained increasing notoriety as a key player in the pathogenesis of atherosclerosis. As atherosclerosis is the commonest cause of vasculogenic erectile dysfunction, in particular in older men, it is frequently considered another manifestation of vascular disease. The risk factors for the development of endothelial dysfunction leading to coronary artery disease, for example, are similar to the risk factor leading to vasculogenic erectile dysfunction.

Men with underlying diseases leading to vascular abnormalities such as diabetes have dysfunctional neurogenic and endothelium-dependent penile smooth muscle relaxation that result in erectile dysfunction. On a cellular level, there may be impairment of the L-arginine NO pathway at a number of sites. While the precise mechanisms have not been clearly defined, endothelial damage may either decrease basal release of NO, or may lead to increased breakdown. Furthermore, eNOS activity may be attenuated by accumulation of NOS inhibitors. In addition to endothelial alterations, vascular smooth muscle cells appear to have a blunted response to nitric oxide. Endothelial function may also be related to microalbuminuria, which appears to influence endothelium-dependent and independent vasodilation. Men with type-2 diabetes mellitus have impaired vasodilation in response to both endothelium-dependent and independent agonists and increased generation of reactive oxygen species that damage endothelial cells either directly or indirectly via effects on lipid peroxidation and by scavenging nitric oxide to produce peroxynitrite (which is a potent oxidant). Other mechanisms leading to endothelial dysfunction are peripheral and autonomic neuropathy, decreased release of acetylcholine by cholinergic nerves, and sparse penile noradrenergic nervous innervation (Rodriguez 2005).

a. Hypertension

The hallmarks of primary hypertension are increased peripheral sympathetic activity, increased vasoconstrictor tone, and decreased endothelium-dependent vasodilation. Some cases of hypertension-associated endothelial dysfunction may be related to eNOS gene variations. Changes in the cyclooxygenase pathway also appear to play a major role, as increased cyclooxygenase activity can lead to an increase in reactive oxygen species, with further disruption of normal endothelial activity. It should be emphasized that dysfunctional endothelium-dependent vasodilation is not merely a cause of hypertension; it exists in several disease states and the degree of endothelial dysfunction does not correlate with blood pressure values.

Hypertension, however, plays an etiologic role in the development of male sexual dysfunction beyond its correlation with endothelial dysfunction. Structural alterations with vascular and corporal remodeling occur that reduce vasodilatory capacity.

b. Dyslipidemia

Hypercholesterolemia has a well-established link to endothelial dysfunction, with oxidized low-density lipoprotein being a key mediator. In familial hypercholesterolemia, endothelial dysfunction is seen prior to clinical arterial disease. Even in the setting of angiographically normal coronary arteries, reduced endothelium-derived NO bioavailability has been seen in the setting of hypercholesterolemia. Endothelial dysfunction is not only related to LDL concentration, but also to LDL size, with smaller particles being associated with such dysfunction. The effects of hypertriglyceridemia, however, are less clear.

c. Obesity

Disturbed endothelial function has been seen in both resistance and conductance arteries of the obese patient, independent of other vascular comorbidities. One mechanism may be the apparent relationship between obesity and a chronic inflammatory state. Elevated levels of the circulating intercellular adhesion molecules–1 (ICAM–1), vascular adhesion molecule (VCAM–1), E and P selectins, tumor necrosis factor alpha (TNFa) and interleukin 6 (IL–6) have been reported in obese men and women. These cytokines have been demonstrated to influence endothelial function and are key contributors in the early atherogenic process. Additionally, this inflammatory process can be a source of oxidative stress, leading to free radical formation and thereby secondarily decreasing NO bioavailability. It has also been suggested that other factors such as oxygen radicals may further contribute to endothelial dysfunction in obesity. Therefore it is not surprising that obesity, especially abdominal obesity, is not only linked to endothelial dysfunction, but also to erectile dysfunction in men.

Men with erectile dysfunction also appear to have impaired endothelial-dependent and independent vasodilation beyond that accounted for by vascular risk factors. Yavuzgil et al. compared brachial artery flow-mediated dilation (FMD) and nitroglycerine-mediated dilation (NMD) in three sets of patients: those with presumed vasculogenic ED and cardiac risk factors, those with similar risk factors but no ED, and a control population without cardiac risk factors or ED (Yavuzgil 2005). They found that brachial artery FMD and NMD were significantly reduced in patients with ED compared to healthy controls. Patients without ED but who had similar risk factors had decreased FMD, but not NMD compared with healthy controls. This suggests impairment in endothelial-independent vasodilation. Other groups also discovered patients with erectile dysfunction to have impaired FMD and NMD compared with controls (Kaiser 2004).

## 2. Cardiovascular diseases in general

Erectile dysfunction is a highly prevalent and increasingly common disorder in men with underlying cardiovascular diseases, since most men with chronic cardiovascular diseases experience decreased libido and decreased frequency of sexual activity, as well as erectile dysfunction. Some unique organic and psychological factors contributing to sexual dysfunction have been identified in patients with underlying cardiovascular problems. Certain risk factors are common to the development of coronary artery disease, heart failure and erectile dysfunction including diabetes mellitus, hypertension, smoking and dyslipidemia (which mostly lead to endothelial dysfunction, see above). Patients with coronary atherosclerosis (arteries diseased by cholesterol plaque build up) are highly likely to have diseased arteries outside of the heart. If the arteries supplying blood to the penis are sufficiently diseased, this can prevent adequate achievement or maintenance of an erection, which sometimes is called "penile angina". Besides potential changes in the pudendal arteries in the penis, stenoses of the common iliac, the hypogastric artery, which supplies the inguinal region with blood in men with peripheral atherosclerosis can lead to erectile dysfunction. Improving blood flow regionally in these patients, either by means of drugs such as PDE–5 inhibitors or by interventional or surgical techniques, have been shown to result in improvement of sexual dysfunction in some cases.

After myocardial infarction many men develop fear that a subsequent cardiac event can be triggered by certain phenomena such as stress, anxiety or others that are combined with an increase of endogenous catecholamines, including sexual activity. This leads to the finding that approximately one third of men cease all sexual activity initially after myocardial infarction, and several do not resume prior sexual activity due to fear of an infarction or even sudden cardiac death. In contrast, less than 1% of all heart attacks occur during sexual activity, and the actual rate of sudden death during sexual activity is very low (around 0.3% of all cases of sudden cardiac death).

Recent data suggest that 75–80% of men with heart failure in different stages suffer from sexual dysfunction, independent on the etiology of the heart disease. (Schwarz 2005, Schwarz 2006)

## 3. Diabetes

Many males with diabetes are impotent, and erectile dysfunction can manifest as an early sign of diabetes. The following are recent statistics demonstrated by the Erectile Dysfunction Institute (EDI):

males with diabetes are two to five times more likely to develop erectile dysfunction than men without the disease. McCulloch et al. (1980) recognized that ED increased progressively with age, from 6% in 20–24 years of age to 52% in men 55–59 year-old. Men with diabetes develop impotence about 10–15 years sooner than men without diabetes. More than fifty percent of men develop diabetic impotence within ten years of getting diabetes. Fifty to sixty percent of diabetic men over age fifty have erectile problems. Fifty to seventy of all diabetic men will experience some degree of erectile difficulties. Men with type–1 diabetes may experience erectile dysfunction at an earlier age since they typically have the disease for a longer period of time. Men with type–2 diabetes, may experience problems later in life. As mentioned, in order for a man to achieve an erection, he must have healthy nerves and blood vessels. In males, diabetes can cause hardening and narrowing of the blood vessels that supply the erectile tissue of the penis, which can directly hamper the process of achieving an erection. Diabetes can also damage the nerves that innervate erectile tissue. The penis can also be less firm during an erection. For men with diabetes, adequate blood glucose control is paramount in preventing/treating their erectile disorder. When diabetes is well controlled, there is diminished risk of the development of any or other secondary complications including erectile dysfunction. Additionally, good blood pressure control, and ceasing the use of tobacco and alcohol can also help diabetic patients in preventing sexual dysfunction.

The use of Phosphodiesterase–5 inhibitors particularly Sildenafil (Viagra) has been implicated in the treatment of all causes of erectile dysfunction, especially diabetes. This drug stimulates blood flow to the penis and along with the other PDE–5 inhibitors (Vardenafil and Tadalfil) is often the first line of treatment of impotence. Viagra however fails in about thirty to forty percent of males who use it. Since diabetes can potentially damage peripheral vascular system, Viagra or any other of the PDE–5 inhibitors may not be a treatment option. In the group of diabetic males who do not benefit from PDE–5 inhibitor therapy, treatments such as penile implants, vacuum devices, drug injections, and urethral suppositories have shown to be successful in treating erectile dysfunction.

Implants have been used for decades and have shown to be quite effective in treating ED. They have been modified over a twenty-five year period and since its advent, approximately 300,000 males have had the procedure for treating their erectile difficulties. Drugs such as alprostadil, papavarine, and phentolamine have been used in injection therapy. These medications act to relax penile muscle tissue thereby promoting blood flow to the penis. Vacuum erection devices draw blood into the penis, and elastic band is placed around the base of the penis in order to preserve the erection. Topical medications including creams rubbed on the skin of the penis and pellets (containing the medication alprostadil) the placed in the tip of the urethra have shown promise in treating erectile dysfunction. Vascular surgery has shown to be effective in improving blood flow to the penis and correcting leaking veins which prevent the male from having an erection (Montague et al. 2005).

## 4. Prostate cancer

Prostate cancer and surgical and medical interventions for the treatment of prostate cancer can all lead to erectile dysfunction. A cancerous prostate can impede nerve impulses and blood flow to the penis, which consequently leads to ED. Erectile difficulties can indeed be one of the first signs of prostate cancer.

Distinct treatments for eradicating prostatic cancer can also lead to ED. A radical prostatectomy that completely removes the prostate can destroy nervous tissue surrounding the prostate that aid in the male's ability to achieve an erection. Even though surgeons strive to preserve the nerve bundles surrounding the prostate, it is never guaranteed that during the operation all of the nerve bundles will be preserved and remain intact. It has been demonstrated that when the surgeon was able to spare part or all of the nerves, trauma per se from the procedure caused some difficulty with erectile function for the first year following the operation. Studies have shown that men who were able to achieve firm erections prior to surgery were less likely to develop ED. Unfortunately, 50–80% of men who undergo a radical prostatectomy become impotent.

Radiation therapy can also lead to ED by directly damaging arteries that carry blood to the penis or lead to the formation of scar tissue (fibrosis) near the prostate which can affect blood flow to the penile tissue. ED as a result of radiation therapy usually does not develop as rapidly as with radical prostatectomy, and may not be apparent for years.

Hormone therapy utilized in the treatment of prostate cancer has shown to lead to ED as early as two to four weeks following the initiation of treatment and is usually accompanied with a loss of sex drive. Hormone therapy is aimed at decreasing the level of androgens specifically testosterone. Sildenafil, intracavernous injection therapy, and penile implants have all been used with some success in the treatment of patients who have received treatment for prostate cancer (Levine 2004).

5. Neurologic (spinal) disorders

Spinal cord injuries can impede or reduce nerve impulses from the brain to the penis and erectile dysfunction may range from partial to complete. Pelvic injuries also harm nerves that innervate the penis and lead to ED. Some studies have shown that frequent bicycling may lead to erectile difficulties. It has been hypothesized that the bicycle seat compresses the path of blood to the penis.

Multiple sclerosis, a disease where cells of the body's immune system attack the outer insulating nerve sheath, can cause the production of scar tissue in random spots through out the central nervous system. The fibrotic tissue formed can then interfere and affect the propagation of nerve impulses to the penis thereby causing ED.

6. Peyronie's disease

Often referred to as penile curvature, Peyronie's disease (PD), which afflicts 3% of the male population, can lead to incomplete erection and erectile dysfunction. This condition usually occurs between the age forty five and sixty. While the average age for contracting PD is fifty, it can occur in men as young as eighteen. Peyronie's disease is characterized by the presence of hardened and calcified tissue (plaque) in the *tunica albuginea* of the penis. This sheath encompasses the spongy tissue of the penis. Peyronie's disease has three main symptoms: lumps present in the penis, pain, and curvature of the penis during erection. Not all causes of Peyronie's disease are known, but physicians agree that sudden trauma to the penis, or vigorous sexual activity can lead to this condition. This disease itself can lead to psychological or physical erectile dysfunction. Regardless of the cause, treatment is available and can be quite successful in alleviating erectile difficulties secondary to Peyronie's disease. Sildenafil, penile implants, vacuum devices, injection therapy, and urethral suppositories all have been used to treat ED due to this condition. Specifically, penile implants have been very useful in treating ED in these patients.

## V. Orgasmic Disorders Due to General Medical Conditions

According to the DSM-IV-TR, female orgasmic disorder is characterized by persistent or recurrent delay in, or absence of orgasm following normal sexual excitement such that a clinician judges the orgasmic capacity to be less than reasonable for age, sexual experience, and adequacy of stimulation. This includes the inability to achieve orgasm through sex with a partner or masturbation.

### A. Female Orgasmic Disorder

Most often this condition is caused by sexual inexperience by one or both partners. Commonly, it is due to lack of adequate clitoral or vaginal stimulation, but it may be due to psychological factors, chronic physical conditions, or medications. Specifically, endocrine diseases such as hypothyroidism, diabetes, and hyperprolactinemia can affect a woman's ability to achieve an orgasm (Sadock 2004).

### B. Male Orgasmic Disorder

The physiological causes of male orgasmic disorder can be due to surgical procedures such as prostatectomy or any type of genitourinary interventions. Any neurological disorders involving the lumbosacral spine and referred pain and paresthesia to the external genitalia can affect a man's ability to orgasm (i.e. pelvic pain syndrome).

### C. Premature Ejaculation rarely has a physical cause, however, neurological disorder, prostatitis (inflammation of the prostate), or urethritis (inflammation of the urethra) can be among the causes. Therefore,

treating the underlying cause can alleviate this particular difficulty. Low doses of the class of the antidepressant class of selective serotonin reuptake inhibitors can be successfully utilized in treating males with premature ejaculation regardless of the underlying physical cause.

## VI. Sexual Pain Disorders Due to General Medical Conditions

### A. Dyspareunia

Pain during intercourse can significantly affect an individual's ability to take pleasure in sex and in many instances may lead to anxiety and depression which in turn can deter and discourage the person from engaging in sexual activity. Careful examination and observation is essential by the physician in order to detect causes that can be readily treated. As defined by the DSM-IV, dyspareunia is characterized by persistent or recurrent genital pain occurring in men or women before, during, or after intercourse. The disturbance should cause marked distress, and can also be characterized by acquired, life long, situational, generalized, due to psychological or combined factors. Dyspareunia should not be diagnosed if an organic cause for the pain has been discovered. In a national survey conducted in 1999 and published in *JAMA*, 7% of women in the study reported pain during intercourse. About 30% of surgical interventions of the female genitalia will result in temporary dyspareunia (Sadock, 2003). Dyspareunia may have several causes. Conditions affecting the skin in the area of the vagina can lead to pain during intercourse. Women with viral or vaginal fungal infections have reported painful sex. Sometimes pain is sensed when the penis enters the vagina and the woman feels that the penis is bumping into something. The uterus may hurt if there is a fibroid growth in the female reproductive tract. Infections of the ovaries or surgeries may leave scar tissue which in turn, can lead to pain. The following gynecological conditions have shown to be responsible for pain before, during, or after intercourse:

1. Cystitis—This is inflammation of the bladder. This condition can lead to painful sex, and women should try to urinate immediately after intercourse to avoid urinary tract infections.

2. Vaginitis—This condition refers to the inflammation of vaginal tissue. Its causes may be due to bacteria or irritants. Women

experiencing this condition secondary to pelvic inflammatory disease usually complain of painful intercourse. Treatment of the underlying cause is necessary to eradicate pain.

3. Urethritis—This is inflammation of the urethra due to urinary tract infection which can result in painful sex. As with cystitis, treatment of underlying cause in this case antibiotics should alleviate any pain.

4. Genital herpes—The herpetic lesions may cause discomfort and pain during intercourse.

5. Genital warts—These warts caused by the Human Papilloma Virus can make sexual activity painful depending on the location. Treatment is through ablative surgery or cryotherapy.

6. Endometriosis—In this condition, there is abnormal uterine tissue growth in distinct parts of the body (ovaries are the most common site). Endometriosis can lead to abnormal bleeding, inflammation, scarring, pain, fatigue, and infertility. The pain can usually manifest when the uterus contracts during orgasm. Treatments include hormone therapy, pain medications, pregnancy, and surgical interventions. Women with this disease should position themselves on top during intercourse to control the amount of penile penetration.

7. Cystocele—This condition occurs when the bladder bulges or herniates into a woman's vagina leading to painful intercourse. Surgical intervention is usually needed to correct this anomaly.

8. Uterine prolapse—This occurs when the uterus falls or "slides" from its normal position into the vaginal canal. The resulting shift in position may lead to painful intercourse.

9. Rectal disease (cancer)—complications such as pain can occur due to the close proximity of the rectum (posterior) to the vagina.

## B. Vaginismus

One out of every one hundred women may suffer from vaginismus. This condition occurs when there is an involuntary muscle constriction of the outer third of the vagina that interferes with penile insertion and intercourse. This response may occur even during routine gynecological examinations when involuntary vaginal constriction prevents the introduction of the speculum into the vagina (Sadock 2004). Even though vaginismus is primarily due to psychological factors, numerous treatment modalities have been established and are currently being studied in order to treat/cure this condition.

About 10% of women with vaginismus are not treated by standard treatments such as lubricants, anesthetic creams, anti-anxiety medications or Kegel exercises. Conventional treatments of females with vaginismus consists mainly of teaching the patient muscle relaxation exercises by having the patient alternate contracting and relaxing the pelvic muscles around the examiner's finger. Some females with this condition can achieve vaginal dilatation by using dilators with increasing diameter or commercial tampons. These instruments are placed in the vagina twice daily for a period of fifteen minutes. Once the diameter of the dilator matches the size of the partner's penis, penetration with the penis can commence.

Iranian researchers, Drs. Shirin Ghazizadeh and M. Nikzad of the Vali-e-Asr Reproductive Health Reseach Center in Tehran have shown that local injections of the botulinum toxin (Botox) is a safe and effective way of treating vaginismus that has been unresponsive to other treatments. The physicians tested a cohort of twenty four women with severe vaginismus that had not been cured with previous treatments (unknown if psychotherapy was utilized as a treatment option). The women were then injected in three sites in muscles on either side of the vagina under light sedation. The participants were followed up a week later, and then for up to twenty four months after the treatment. Eighteen of the twenty three patients (one patient dropped out) were successfully able to have intercourse following the first injection. Four patients reported some pain with intercourse, and one reported to be cured following a second series of injections. Interestingly, none of the patients experienced a return of vaginismus (Ghazizadeh & Nikzad 2004).

Pain during intercourse in males has not been well studied. It has been associated with Peyronie's disease where sclerotic plaques invade the sheath which covers the penis. Pelvic pain syndrome (Prostatodynia) has also been associated with painful erection, ejaculation, and pain during intercourse. No current definitive treatments are available for alleviating the pain associated with prostatodynia. The cause of this condition remains unknown, even though some physicians consider local trauma to the penis and external genitalia or vigorous sexual activity as potential risks for developing pelvic pain syndrome. Some patients have benefited from monthly prostatic massage from their urologists, sitz baths, herbal medications (i. e. Graminex), and acupuncture.

## Conclusion

Sexual dysfunction, while rarely threatening to physical well being, can exert a heavy psychological toll on an individual. It can affect one's sense of general well being and quality of life. Sexual difficulties as illustrated can be caused by both psychological and physical factors/conditions. The aim of this chapter is to introduce the most common general medical conditions which can potentially lead to any of the four major sexual disorders namely: disorder of desire, arousal, orgasm, and pain with intercourse. It was also illustrated that with the appropriate diagnosis and treatment of the underlying cause, one can restore normal sexual functioning to ensure a more enjoyable life. Our goal is to educate specifically people who have medical conditions which can potentially hamper their sexual functioning, and encourage them to not only optimize their self care, but also to seek help as soon as possible.

## *References*

Abramov LA. Sexual life and sexual frigidity among women developing acute myocardial infarction. Psychosom Med 38: 418–25, 1976

American Psychiatric Association (APA): Diagnostic and Statistical Manual of Mental Disorders. 4th ed. Text Revision. Washington, DC, American Psychiatric Publishing Inc, 2000

Bachmann GA, Leiblum SR: The impact of hormones on menopausal sexuality: a literature review. Menopause 11(1):120–130, 2004

Basson R: The complexities of female sexual arousal disorder: potential role of pharmacotherapy World Journal of Urology 20;119–126, 2002

Braunstein GD, Sundwall DA, Katz M, Shifren JL, Buster JE, Simon JA, Bachman G, Aguirre OA, Lucas JD, Rodenberg C, Buch A, Watts NB: Safety and efficacy of a testosterone patch for the treatment of hypoactive sexual desire disorder in surgically menopausal women: a randomized, placebo-controlled trial. Arch Intern Med. 165(14):1571–2, 2005

Ghazizadeh S, Nikzad M: Botulinum Toxin in the Treatment of Refractory Vaginismus. Obstetrics & Gynecology 104:922–925, 2004

Golombok S, Rust J, Pickard C: Sexual problems encountered in general practice. Br J Sex Med 11:171–5, 1984

Kaiser DR, Billups K, Mason C, Wetterling R, Lundberg JL, Bank AJ. Impaired Brachial Artery Endothelium-Dependent and –Independent Vasodilation in Men With Erectile Dysfunction and No Other Clinical Cardiovascular Disease. J Am Coll Cardiol 43:179–84, 2004

Levine LA: Erectile Dysfunction following Treatment of Prostate Canaer; New insights and Theraputic Options J Men's Health Gend 1(4); 328–333, 2004

McCulloch DK, Campbell IW, Wu FC, Prescott RJ, Clarke BF. The prevalence of diabetic impotence. Diabetologia 18:279–283,1980

Montague, D.K., J.P. Jarow, G.A. Broderick, R.R. Dmochowski, J.P. Heaton, T.F. Lue, et al.: The management of erectile dysfunction: an AUA update. J Urol. 174(1): 230–9, 2005

Rodriguez JJ, Al Dashti R, Schwarz ER. Linking erectile dysfunction and coronary artery disease, Int J Impot Res 17 (Suppl 1):S12–8, 2005

Sadock VA : Normal Human Sexuality and Sexual and Gender Identity Disorders In Kaplan and Sadock Comprehensive Textbook of Psychiatry, 8th edition, Sadock BJ & Sadock VA, Editors. Lippincott Williams & Wilkins, Baltimore, Maryland, 2004

Schwarz ER, Rodriguez JJ. Sex and the heart. Int J Impot Res 17, Suppl. 1, S4–6, 2005

Schwarz ER, Rasatogi S, Kapur V, Sulemanjee N, Rodriguez JJ. Erectile dysfunction in heart failure patients. J Am Coll Cardiol, in press, 2006

Vacanti LJ, Caramelli, B. Age and psychologic disorders. Variables associated to post-infarction sexual dysfunction. Arg Bras Cardiol 85: 110–4, 2005.

Yavuzgil O, Altay B, Zoghi M, Gurgun C, Kayikcioglu M, Kultursay H. Endothelial function in patients with vasculogenic erectile dysfunction. Int J of Cardiol 103:19–26, 2005

# 5

# Sexual Desire Disorders

Waguih William IsHak, M.D.
Aelred Boyle, M.D.

## I. Introduction

In 1979 Helen Singer Kaplan was the first to identify sexual desire as a component of the sexual response cycle (see Chapter 1) after treating and evaluating nearly 6,000 patients using a biopsychosocial approach and psychodynamically oriented sex therapy. Kaplan's sequential model of human sexual response places desire before arousal (Kaplan, 1995). Walter Everaerd and Ellen Laan (2001) argued that the Human Sexual Response Model as a sequential model places desire before arousal. However, desire could be part of arousal when it is triggered by a sexual stimulus and facilitated or inhibited by situational and sexual partner variables.

Stephen Levine said that sexual desire is "a slippery concept" since it is the sum of forces that drive people close to and away from sexual behavior. He viewed desire as consisting of drive (biological), motive (individual and relationship psychology), and wish (cultural) components. Age, gender, social situation, health and opposing components (e.g., drive and motive being unsynchronized) will therefore affect sexual desire (Levine 2003). More recently, Basson, et al. (2004) highlighted the issue that desire and arousal can be concurrent.

According to the DSM-IV-TR (APA 2000) sexual desire disorders are divided into two categories: sexual aversion disorder and hypoactive sexual desire disorder. Women's sexual desire disorders are also discussed in Chapter 10 on Women's Sexual Health.

### Hypoactive Sexual Desire Disorder

Persistently or recurrently deficient (or absent) sexual fantasies and desire for sexual activity resulting in marked distress or interpersonal difficulty while it is not better accounted for by another Axis I disorder (apart from other sexual disorders). The judgment of deficiency or absence is made by the clinician, taking into account factors that affect sexual functioning, such as age and the context of the person's life.

### Sexual Aversion Disorder

Persistent or recurrent extreme aversion to, and avoidance of, all (or almost all) genital sexual contact with a sexual partner resulting in marked distress or interpersonal difficulty while it is not better accounted for by another Axis I disorder (apart from other sexual disorders).

### Other Sexual Desire Disorders

It is important to note that the DSM-IV does not have a separate category for increased sexual desire or activity since the empirical evidence is still lacking for the need for such a category. However, this chapter will cover briefly some of the information available on this issue.

## II. Hypoactive Sexual Desire Disorder (HSDD)

### A. Criteria

Table 1 shows the DSM-IV-TR criteria for this disorder. The clinician gauges the deficiency taking into account the person's life situation and age.

**TABLE 1**
**DSM-IV Diagnostic Criteria for**
**302.71 Hypoactive Sexual Desire Disorder**

A. Persistently or recurrently deficient (or absent) sexual fantasies and desire for sexual activity. The judgment of deficiency or absence is made by the clinician, taking into account factors that affect sexual functioning, such as age and the context of the person's life.

B. The disturbance causes marked distress or interpersonal difficulty.

C. The sexual dysfunction is not better accounted for by another Axis I disorder (except another Sexual Dysfunction) and is not due exclusively to the direct physiological effects of a substance (e.g., a drug of abuse, a medication) or a general medical condition.

Specify type:  Lifelong Type
                Acquired Type
Specify type:  Generalized Type
                Situational Type
Specify:       Due to Psychological Factors
                Due to Combined Factors

Reprinted with permission from the Diagnostic and Statistical Manual of Mental Disorders, Fourth Edition, Text Revision. Copyright 2000 American Psychiatric Association

B. **Epidemiology**

In the United States, the National Health and Social Life Survey revealed that lack of sexual desire is the most common sexual complaint in women and estimated that approximately 33% of women experience a lack of sexual interest or desire at some point in their lives (Laumann et al. 1999). Low sexual desire increases with age in both genders (Basson et al., 2004). This may be due in part to a declining bioavailability (quantity available for biological use) of sex steroids. Twenty-six percent of men over 70 have a decrease in bioavailable testosterone compared to younger men (Panser et al. 1995).

C. **Etiology**

1. **Biological factors:** when a medical or substance etiology for hypoactive sexual desire is found, the disorder is not diagnosed if the condition resolves with treatment of the underlying condition.

a. General medical conditions: anemia, hypertension, diabetes mellitus, thyroid dysfunction, multiple sclerosis, systemic lupus erythematosus, traumatic brain injury, HIV infection, changes in sex hormones, or polycystic ovary syndrome (PCOS): (see section II.E.1.c.) The impact of these medical illnesses (and/or their complications or treatment) could contribute further to sexual dysfunction, e.g. PCOS may be associated with hirsutism, which might affect body image and self-esteem. Treatment of this condition using anti-androgens might lead to further dysfunction.

b. Substances: multiple drugs can cause sexual dysfunction but especially suspect are selective serotonin reuptake inhibitor antidepressants, first generation antipsychotics, diuretics, beta receptor blocking antihypertensives ("beta-blockers"), anti-androgens, and substances of abuse including alcohol.

2. Psychological factors:

a. All psychiatric disorders can decrease sexual desire, especially depression and anxiety.

b. Sexual trauma, such as incest, sexual abuse, molestation, or rape

c. Dyspareunia and negative sexual experiences

3. Social factors:

a. Relationship factors: e.g. conflicts, anger, lack of trust

b. Stressors: financial, employment, family problems, caring for young children.

   According to the Canadian Society of Obstetricians and Gynaecologists, the most commonly observed reasons for low libido in women are tension-fatigue states and relationship difficulties.

## D. Pathophysiology

Sexual desire is affected by levels of sex steroids (estrogen and testosterone), and neurotransmitters, such as dopamine and serotonin. Stoleru et al. (2003) used PET scans to study the brains of men with HSDD compared to normal controls. During exposure to visual sexual stimuli, HSDD patients had abnormally maintained activity in the medial orbitofrontal cortex, an area that may be involved in inhibiting motivated behavior. Activation in control subjects and deactivation or unchanged activity in patients with HSDD were found in the secondary somatosensory cortex and inferior parietal lobules (regions mediating emotional and motor imagery processes), as well as in the premotor processing areas of the anterior cingulate gyrus and frontal lobes. However whether these changes are causes or consequences of HSDD is not yet known.

## E. Treatment Approaches

### 1. Diagnostic work-up:

a. If the patient has a partner, interview the patient both individually and with the partner to gather as much information as possible, including information about issues in the relationship.

b. Physical exam and medical history to identify general medical problems and effects of substances.

c. Standard and specialized laboratory testing: levels of dihydroepiandrosterone-sulfate (DHEA-S), free or bioavailable testosterone (the equilibrium dialysis method is the most reliable for free), SHBG (sex hormone binding globulin), estrone or estradiol, FSH (follicle stimulating hormone, prolactin, TSH (thyroid stimulating hormone) and ferritin. Consider referral to an endocrinologist.

d. Psychiatric evaluation to rule out psychiatric disorders, especially bipolarity, depression and anxiety disorders (see Appendix 3).

e. Assessment instruments (rating scales) can be useful to assess both baseline functioning and progress (Davis 1998):

Spector, Carey and Steinberg Sexual Desire Inventory

Hurlbert Index of Sexual Desire

Sexual Experience Scale by Frenken and Vennix

### 2. Biological treatments:

a. General: discontinuation or substitution of medications causing decreased sexual desire is sometimes effective.

b. Physical: self-exploration, stimulation and masturbation have been recommended for both women and men with HSDD as ways to become comfortable with sexual feelings and increase desire.

c. Medications:

1) PDE–5 inhibitors: there is little evidence to show that sildenafil citrate (Viagra) increases sexual desire (as opposed to arousal) in either men or women although small studies showed it effective in reversing SSRI-induced loss of sexual desire.

2) Estrogens and progestins were reviewed by Robinson et al. (2003): a 3 to 6 month trial off of oral contraceptives or replacing oral contraceptives with triphasic oral contraceptives may be helpful for some patients. Peri- or post-menopausal patients may benefit from transdermal HT (hormone therapy). Estrogen in any form (e.g., transdermal patch, vaginal ring, vaginal cream) with oral progestins may be effective for some.

3) Testosterone: testosterone supplementation in postmenopausal women (natural or surgical menopause, i.e., post-oophorectomy) seems to be effective. Topical 1% to 2% testosterone ointment can be applied daily to the labia or inner thigh initially, then 1 to 3 times per week (Robinson et al. 2003). Shifren et al. (2000) and others (Simon 2005; Buster 2005, and Braunstein (2005) showed the effectiveness of transdermal testosterone in women post oophorectomy. Oral methyltestosterone can be used as a sole agent or in combination with estrogen but carries the risk of lowering HDL cholesterol. Testosterone patches and gel are showing some promising results in investigatory clinical trials. More studies are needed to assess the effectiveness of testosterone in premenopausal women.

4) Bupropion sustained or extended release (Wellbutrin SR or Wellbutrin XL): Seagraves et al. (2001), in a study of 51 non-depressed women, reported that 29% responded to bupropion 150 mg bid as early as two weeks after beginning treatment.

5) Other antidepressants: treatment of underlying depression and anxiety can improve low sexual desire. Antidepressants with

the lowest risk of causing sexual dysfunction should obviously be chosen, e.g., bupropion, or mirtazapine. Tricyclic antidepressants tend to cause less sexual dysfunction than SSRIs.

    6) Herbal treatments: these are discussed in Chapter 9 on Alternative Medicine in Sexual Performance Enhancement.

  d. No recommended surgical treatment exists for HSDD.

**3. Psychosocial treatments:**

  a. General: including the partner, when there is one, in the assessment and treatment achieves the best outcome.

  b. Psychodynamic psychotherapy: individual sessions to make conscious any underlying conflicts about sex.

  c. Individual or group cognitive behavioral therapy (CBT).

  d. Behavioral therapy, biofeedback.

  e. Couples therapy and sex therapy to address interpersonal and communication problems.

  f. Interpersonal psychotherapy to identify fears and guilt. Psychotherapy is also essential for the process of recovery from trauma, both sexual and nonsexual.

**4. Communication and education** are an essential part of the treatment plan for patients with HSDD. The patient and/or partner may be in denial or may be feeling rejected, frustrated, angry, anxious, guilty, or depressed.

## F. Prognosis

The prognosis of HSDD is unknown but may be relatively better in highly motivated patients.

# III. Sexual Aversion Disorder

## A. Definition and Phenomenology

Patients with sexual aversion disorder (SAD) are averse to and avoid sexual contact, whereas patients with HSDD have decreased desire for sexual contact.

---

**TABLE 2**
**DSM-IV Diagnostic Criteria for 302.79 Sexual Aversion Disorder**

A. Persistent or recurrent extreme aversion to, and avoidance of, all (or almost all) genital sexual contact with a sexual partner.

B. The disturbance causes marked distress or interpersonal difficulty.

C. The sexual dysfunction is not better accounted for by another Axis I disorder (except another Sexual Dysfunction).

| | |
|---|---|
| Specify type: | Lifelong Type |
| | Acquired Type |
| Specify type: | Generalized Type |
| | Situational Type |
| Specify: | Due to Psychological Factors |
| | Due to Combined Factors |

Reprinted with permission from the Diagnostic and Statistical Manual of Mental Disorders, Fourth Edition, Text Revision. Copyright 2000 American Psychiatric Association

---

SAD patients report anxiety, fear, or disgust in sexual situations and generally avoid them, including touching and kissing. Sufferers may have panic attacks, feel nauseated or dizzy, or pass out.

### B. Epidemiology

There is no clear epidemiological information available for sexual aversion and it is therefore assumed to be a rare disorder but this may be an incorrect assumption. Some studies estimate a 2% prevalence of SAD and report that the disorder is more common in women than men. In the United States, the National Health and Social Life Survey (Laumann et al. 1999) reported that 21% of women found sex not pleasurable, 19% had trouble lubricating, and 14% experienced pain during intercourse, all of which are reported causes of sexual aversion disorder or hypoactive sexual desire disorder. The study excluded 139 men and 238 women who were sexually inactive in the year prior to the survey, which may have biased the results.

### C. Etiology

1. **Biological factors:** biological factors are poorly studied in sexual aversion disorder. More information is available on hypoactive sexual

desire disorder and may be helpful in understanding sexual aversion. Current hypotheses for SAD include low testosterone and serotonin levels.

2. **Psychosocial factors:** possible etiologies or contributors to lifelong SAD include sexual trauma (incest, molestation, sexual abuse, rape), repressive upbringing, rigid religious training, or initial attempts at intercourse that resulted in severe dyspareunia. Situational sexual aversion can be present in relationships with significant conflicts, or where there is a history of sexual trauma or pain. Severe anxiety and avoidance are also seen in persons who attempt to have sexual relations incongruent with their sexual orientation.

   Excessive worry does not appear to be a risk factor for sexual desire problems in non-clinical populations (Katz and Jardine 1999). However, Figueira et al. (2001) reported that sexual aversion disorder was the most common sexual dysfunction in both men (35%) and women (50%) with panic disorder. Raboch and Faltus (1991) reported a higher incidence of SAD in patients with anorexia nervosa. This last finding may be confounded by a higher prevalence of childhood sexual abuse in patients with eating disorders than in those without eating disorders.

## D. Pathophysiology

The pathophysiology of sexual aversion disorder remains poorly understood. Currently it seems that the disorder may be due more to learned experiences than to innate factors.

## E. Treatment Approaches

1. **Diagnostic work-up:**

   a. If the patient has a partner, interview the patient both individually and with the partner to gather as much information as possible, including information about issues in the relationship.

   b. Physical exam and medical history to identify general medical problems and effects of substances.

   c. Medical work-up to rule out general medical problems, and substance-induced effects. For specialized laboratory testing please see section I.E.1.c.

d. Psychiatric evaluation to rule out disorders that might be related to sexual aversion, especially post-traumatic stress disorder (PTSD) and panic disorder.

e. Assessment instruments (rating scales): the Sexual Aversion Scale (SAS) is a 30-item questionnaire based on the DSM-IV criteria for sexual aversion that assesses sexual fears and avoidance (Katz et al. 1989).

2. **Biological treatments:**

Biological treatments are not well studied in SAD. Some of the treatments available for HSDD may be helpful for improving response to psychosocial interventions.

3. **Psychosocial treatments:**

a. General: Including the partner, when there is one, in the assessment and treatment achieves the best outcome.

b. Psychodynamic psychotherapy: individual sessions to make conscious any underlying conflicts about sex.

c. Individual cognitive behavioral therapy (CBT) for anxiety reduction, cognitive restructuring and minimizing avoidance behaviors.

d. Behavioral therapy: desensitization has been effective in several case reports (Finch 2001).

e. Couples therapy and sex therapy to address interpersonal and communication problems.

f. Interpersonal psychotherapy to identify fears and guilt. Psychotherapy is also essential for the process of recovery from trauma, both sexual and nonsexual.

4. **Communication and education** are an essential part of the treatment plan for patients with SAD. The patient and/or partner may be in denial or may be feeling rejected, frustrated, angry, anxious, guilty, or depressed.

## F. Prognosis

The prognosis of SAD is unknown but may be relatively better in highly motivated patients.

## IV. Other Sexual Desire Disorders
## Hyperactive Sexual Desire Disorder

### A. Definition

Increased sexual desire and sexual activity could be labeled as Hyperactive Sexual Desire Disorder (Leiblum and Rosen, 1988), which is not a DSM-IV category. Manifestations of this behavior include excessive masturbation, increased engagement in sexual intercourse, pornography, and online or computer-based sexual activities. It is well documented that there is an increased sexual desire in patients with Bipolar Disorder, Cyclothymia and Schizoaffective Disorder during manic and hypomanic episodes. Disinhibition (behavioral and sexual) is also found in patients with dementia, delirium, and medical illnesses, e.g., frontal lobe tumors, epilepsy, and traumatic brain injury. Increased sexual behavior was described in Kluver-Bucy syndrome (Sadock et al. 1997). Alcohol, illicit drugs, and prescription medications such as dopamine agonists were implicated in increased desire and increased sexual activity.

### B. Models of Understanding This Disorder

Gold and Heffner (1998) reported on three models used to describe hyperactive sexual desire:

1. The addiction model postulates that sex can become a substance of addiction since patients report withdrawal, tolerance, and spending large amounts of time looking for sex, engaging in sex, or recovering from its effects. They also report impairment of functioning and legal, financial, and medical consequences (Carnes 1983). Support for this model also includes the fact that some patients have been successfully treated using 12-step self-help groups (such as Sexual Compulsives Anonymous: SCA—see IV.C.2 below), which are based on the 12-step groups of Alcoholics Anonymous (AA). Cognitive behavioral therapy has also proven effective for some (Carnes and Adams 2002).

2. The compulsive model hypothesizes that sexual thoughts, images or impulses can become obsessive in intensity for some people and that this can lead to compulsive, repetitive engagement in sexual

activity to reduce anxiety. Many authors use the terms sex addiction and sexual compulsivity interchangeably (Quadland 1985). Support for this model comes from successful treatment courses using high doses of SSRIs or clomipramine which treat obsessions and compulsions and cause sexual dysfunction. It remains unclear whether the medication effectiveness was due to serotonin reuptake inhibition or due to the side effect of decreased sexual desire.

3. The impulse control disorder model is the newest model and is based on viewing the desire for sex (in those with hyperactive sexual activity) as an impulse (like pathological gambling or pyromania) that is extinguished by engaging in excessive repeated sexual activity followed by significant remorse (Barth and Kinder 1987). Support for this model comes from studies showing high co-morbidity of compulsive sexual behavior and impulse control disorders, and also from response to high doses of SSRIs.

## C. Treatment Approaches

1. Biological: fluoxetine 60–80 mg per day, fluvoxamine 100–200 mg per day, clomipramine 150–300 mg per day. There are case reports of naltrexone being effective, especially at the higher end of the dose range of 150 mg per day (Grant and Kim 2001, Raymond 2002).

2. Psychosocial: group psychotherapy, individual cognitive behavioral therapy, behavioral therapy, and self-help groups (Sex Addicts Anonymous, Sexaholics Anonymous, Sex and Love Addicts Anonymous, Sexual Compulsives Anonymous, S-Anon for family members, etc.).

## V. Conclusion and Future Directions

Hypoactive Sexual Desire Disorder (HSDD) is the most common sexual disorder in women. Sexual Aversion Disorder appears to be rare but little research is available on its prevalence, and its sufferers may be avoiding clinical attention. Desire problems need to be fully evaluated and treated using a biopsychosocial approach. Further studies on the effects of hormones and other biomedical interventions are needed. Investigation of hyperactive sexual desire is warranted to evaluate whether or not this is indeed a legitimate disorder.

## *References*

American Psychiatric Association (APA): Diagnostic and Statistical Manual of Mental Disorders. 4th ed. Text Revision Washington, DC: American Psychiatric Publishing Inc, 2000

Barth RJ. Kinder BN: The mislabeling of sexual impulsivity. Journal of Sex & Marital Therapy 13(1):15–23, 1987

Basson, Althof, Davis, et al. Summary of the recommendations on sexual dysfunction in women. Journal of Sexual Medicine. 1(1):24–34, 2004

Carnes PJ and Adams KM: Clinical management of sex addiction, New York: Brunner-Routledge, 2002Carnes, Patrick: Out of the shadows: understanding sexual addiction, Center City, MN : Hazelden Information & Edu, 1983

Davis CM; Yarber WL; Bauserman R; Schreer G; & Davis SL. (Eds.): Handbook of sexuality-related measures. Thousand Oaks, Calif., Sage Publ., 1998

Everaerd Walter, Laan Ellen and Both Stephanie (editors): Sexual Appetite, Desire and Motivation: Energetics of the Sexual System. Amsterdam, Netherlands: Knaw Edita, 2001

Figueira I, Possidente E, Marques C, Hayes K: Sexual dysfunction: a neglected complication of panic disorder and social phobia. Archives of Sexual Behavior 30(4):369–77, 2001

Finch S: Sexual aversion disorder treated with behavioural desensitization. Canadian Journal of Psychiatry—Revue Canadienne de Psychiatrie. 46(6):563–4, 2001

Gold SN. Heffner CL. Sexual addiction: many conceptions, minimal data. Clinical Psychology Review 18(3):367–81, 1998

Grant JE, Kim SW: A case of kleptomania and compulsive sexual behavior treated with naltrexone. Annals of Clinical Psychiatry 13(4):229–31, 2001

Hensley PL, Nurnberg HG: SSRI sexual dysfunction: a female perspective. Journal of Sex & Marital Therapy 28 Suppl 1:143–53, 2002

Kaplan, Helen Singer: Disorders of sexual desire and other new concepts and techniques in sex therapy, New York : Simon and Schuster, 1979

Kaplan, Helen Singer: The Sexual Desire Disorders: Dysfunctional Regulation of Sexual Motivation, New York: Brunner/Mazel, 1995

Katz RC. Gipson MT. Kearl A. Kriskovich M. Assessing sexual aversion in college students: the Sexual Aversion Scale. Journal of Sex & Marital Therapy 15(2):135–40, 1989

Katz RC. Jardine D. The relationship between worry, sexual aversion, and low sexual desire. Journal of Sex & Marital Therapy 25(4):293–6, 1999

Laumann EO, Paik A, Rosen RC: Sexual Dysfunction in the United States: Prevalence and Predictors. JAMA 281:537–544, 1999

Leiblum SR and Rosen RC: Sexual desire disorders. New York: Guilford, 1988

Levine SB: The nature of sexual desire: a clinician's perspective. Archives of Sexual Behavio. 32(3):279–85, 2003

Panser LA, Rhodes A, Girman CJ, et al.: Sexual function of men ages 40 to 79 years: The Olmsted County Study of Urinary Symptoms and Health Status among Men. J Am Geriatr Soc 43:1107–1111, 1995

Quadland MC. Compulsive sexual behavior: definition of a problem and an approach to treatment. Journal of Sex & Marital Therapy. 11(2):121–32, 1985

Raboch JS, Faltus F. Sexuality of women with anorexia nervosa. Acta Psychiatr Scand 84:9–11, 1991

Raymond NC, Grant JE, Kim SW. Coleman E: Treatment of compulsive sexual behaviour with naltrexone and serotonin reuptake inhibitors: two case studies. International Clinical Psychopharmacology 17(4):201–5, 2002

Robinson B. Feldman J. Striepe M. Raymond N. Mize S. Women's sexual health: an interdisciplinary approach to treating low sexual desire. Minnesota Medicine. 86(7):34–41, 2003

Sadock VA, IsHak WW, and Rodack V: Hypersexuality: Addiction or Compulsion? Presented at the annual meeting of the American Psychiatric Association, San Diego, May 1997

Segraves RT. Croft H. Kavoussi R. Ascher JA. Batey SR. Foster VJ. Bolden-Watson C. Metz A. Bupropion sustained release (SR) for the treatment of hypoactive sexual desire disorder (HSDD) in nondepressed women. Journal of Sex & Marital Therapy 27(3):303–16, 2001

Shifren JL. Braunstein GD. Simon JA. Casson PR. Buster JE. Redmond GP. Burki RE. Ginsburg ES. Rosen RC. Leiblum SR. Caramelli KE. Mazer NA. Transdermal testosterone treatment in women with impaired sexual function after oophorectomy. New England Journal of Medicine 343(10):682–8, 2000

Simons JS, Carey MP ; Prevalence of sexual dysfunctions: results from a decade of research. ; Arch Sex Behav; 30(2):177–219, 2001

Stoleru S. Redoute J. Costes N. Lavenne F. Bars DL. Dechaud H. Forest MG. Pugeat M. Cinotti L. Pujol JF. Brain processing of visual sexual stimuli in men with hypoactive sexual desire disorder. Psychiatry Research. 124(2):67–86, 2003

Warnock JJ. Female hypoactive sexual desire disorder: epidemiology, diagnosis and treatment. CNS Drugs. 16(11):745–53, 2002

# 6

# Sexual Arousal Disorders

ALBERT A. MIKHAIL, M.D.
JAY YEW, M.D.

## I. Introduction

Contrary to the original works by Hippocrates, who believed erections developed from the combination of pneuma (air) and "vital spirits" flowing to the penis, modern day knowledge has better revealed the male and female response to sexual arousal. This common phenomenon in both men and women is centered at the fact that pelvic vasocongestion takes place leading to the normal response of penile erections in men and vaginal elongation and lubrication along with clitoral erection in women. Sexual arousal disorders occur in both men and women due to an inability to achieve or maintain this pelvic vasocongestion until the completion sexual activity. In men this disorder presents as Male Erectile Disorder while in women, this sexual arousal disorder affects the lubrication-swelling response to sexual excitement.

### Male Erectile Disorder (ED)

ED is defined by the DSM-IV-TR as the inability to attain or to maintain an adequate erection until the completion of the sexual activity resulting in marked distress or interpersonal difficulty while it is not better accounted for by another Axis I disorder (apart from other sexual disorders).

### Female Sexual Arousal Disorder (FSAD)

FSAD is defined by the DSM-IV-TR (APA 2000) as the persistent or recurrent inability to attain or maintain an adequate lubrication-swelling response of sexual excitement until completion of sexual activity resulting in marked distress or interpersonal difficulty while it is not better accounted for by another Axis I disorder (apart from other sexual disorders).

### Other Sexual Arousal Disorders

Atypical syndromes were described in the context of the arousal phase such as repeated yawning during intercourse (reported with SSRIs), severe dissociative symptoms, and increased aggression. These presentations are mostly reported as isolated cases and will not be covered in this chapter.

## II. Male Erectile Disorder (ED)

### A. Definition and Phenomenology

Male Erectile Disorder (ED) as defined by the DSM-IV-TR is the inability to attain or to maintain an adequate erection until the completion of the sexual activity. This disorder causes marked distress or interpersonal difficulty. The normal physiology of erectile function is a complex process involving the neural and vascular structures of the penis as well as the integrity of the expansile tissue within the penis itself. Several etiologies, organic and inorganic, work independently or in combination to exacerbate ED.

Patients, typically report decreased rigidity of erections and less commonly, total absence of erections. Patients may achieve an erection sufficient for penetration; however, they experience loss of tumescence during penetration or thrusting. Psychosocial etiologies typically involve intact nocturnal and morning erections and commonly present

---

**TABLE 1**

**Diagnostic Criteria for 302.72 Male Erectile Disorder**

A. Persistent or recurrent inability to attain, or to maintain until completion of the sexual activity, an adequate erection.

B. The disturbance causes marked distress or interpersonal difficulty.

C. The Male Erectile Disorder is not better accounted for by another Axis I disorder (other than a Sexual Dysfunction) and is not due exclusively to the direct physiological effects of a substance (e.g., a drug of abuse, a medication) or a general medical condition.

Specify type:  Lifelong Type
　　　　　　　Acquired Type

Specify type:  Generalized Type
　　　　　　　Situational Type

Specify:  Due to Psychological Factors
　　　　　Due to Combined Factors

Reprinted with permission from the Diagnostic and Statistical Manual of Mental Disorders, Fourth Edition, Text Revision. Copyright 2000 American Psychiatric Association

---

with situational Male Erectile Disorder. The various types are: Lifelong Type/Acquired Type, Generalized Type/Situational Type, and Due to Psychological Factors or Due to Combined Factors.

## B. Epidemiology

The prevalence of ED increases with age. The overall prevalence of ED in men ranges from 10–52% (Laumann et al. 1999). When adjusted for age, prevalence is 22% for 50–54 year old men, while in 70–78 year olds; the prevalence increases to 54%. In the Massachusetts Male Aging Study the likelihood of becoming completely impotent tripled from 5% in men 40 years of age to 15% in men 70 years of age (Feldman et al. 1994).

## C. Etiology

### 1. Biological factors:

　　a. General: As outline before, the risk of ED increases with age. Genetic factors were identified in ED. Fischer et al. (2004) studied ED in 890 monozygotic and 619 dizygotic twin pairs. They concluded that the estimated heritability of liability for dysfunction in having an erection is 35% and in maintaining an erection is 42%.

b. Substance-induced ED: alcohol, illicit drugs, prescription and over the counter medications, dietary supplements and herbs in addition to toxins could cause ED. An extensive discussion of substances affecting sexual functioning is presented in Chapter 3 on Substance-induced Sexual Dysfunction.

c. Medical factors include congenital etiologies, neuropathic and vasculopathic sources as well as hormonal imbalances and certain medical conditions.

   1) Congenital anomalies include micropenis, epispadias, and bladder extrophy. Neuropathies may occur in disorders such as multiple sclerosis, multiple system atrophy (Shy-Drager syndrome), spinal cord injury or lower motor neuron injury.

   2) Diabetes Mellitus is also a common cause of neuropathic and vasculogenic ED.

   3) Vascular causes include arterial insufficiency, which may stem from aorto-iliac disease (Leriche syndrome) or from micro vessel disease, atherosclerosis, smoking, or end stage renal disease.

   4) Structural anatomic problems include scarring of the expansile erectile tissue from priapism (prolonged painful erection) as well as vascular abnormalities such as venous leak, fistulae, or arterial-venous shunt after penile trauma.

   5) Endocrine conditions leading to increased prolactin levels also play a role in ED, while hypogonadal states tend to decrease libido and the frequency of nocturnal erections without impairing sexually stimulated erections. Hypogonadism and low testosterone levels are to due to genetic factors, pituitary or hypothalamic abnormalities, malnutrition, Orchitis, Mumps, testicular injuries, radiation, and excessive exercise in athletes.

   6) Pelvic: Patients undergoing pelvic surgery or irradiation are also at risk for the development of ED.

7) Renal: ED is common among renal patients on dialysis. This form of ED improves after successful renal transplantation; however, may also be exacerbated if the internal iliac artery is utilized for graft revascularization.

8) General conditions that have been associated with ED include coronary artery disease, hypertension, hyperlipidemia, peripheral vascular disease, benign prostatic hyperplasia, and morbid obesity.

## 2. Psychosocial factors:

a. Psychiatric Disorders (see Appendix 3): Mood Disorders especially depression, Anxiety Disorders, Psychotic Disorders with or without nihilistic delusions that the penis does not exist. Performance anxiety is known to interfere with ability to obtain and maintain erection.

b. Stressors: traumas, losses, and conflicts in addition to financial, vocational, and residential factors

c. Relational issues such as lack of attractiveness to the partner, relationship conflicts, and lack of adequacy of sexual stimulation.

## D. Pathophysiology

Erection formation begins with parasympathetic nerve stimulation in coordination with nonadrenergic noncholinergic nerves that leads to the release of nitric oxide. Nitric oxide acts by increasing cyclic-guanosine monophosphate (cGMP) levels in cavernosal smooth muscle, which is later metabolized by phosphodiesterases. cGMP activates protein kinase G that results in relaxation of cavernosal smooth muscle. Cavernosal bodies fill with blood compressing small emissary veins against the tunica albuginea layer trapping blood in the corporal bodies under pressure. This accumulation of "trapped" blood causes increased length, girth, and firmness of the penis. Any disruption of this process will contribute to ED.

With increasing age structural changes are noted which contribute to ED. These changes include a decreased ratio of elastic fibers to collagen and a decreased ratio of smooth muscle to connective tissue, which contributes to venous leakage. There is also a decrease in collagen type

3 with simultaneous increase in collagen type–1, which decreases over-all compliance (Seftel 2003).

The penis consists of paired corpora cavernosa, and a ventral corpus spongiosum surrounding the urethra and distally forming the glans penis. A thick fibrous sheath, the tunica albuginea, surrounds each of the corpora cavernosa, and all three corpora are bound together by Buck's fascia. The ischiocavernosus and bulbospongiosus muscles surround the proximal portions of the corpora cavernosa. Each corpus consists of smooth muscle bundles, elastic fibers, collagen, and loose fibrous tissue, which form trabeculae. In between the trabeculae are blood-filled lacunar spaces lined by flat endothelial cells. The arterial supply to the penis consists of the internal pudendal arteries, which become the penile arteries. Each penile artery terminates in bulbar, urethral, dorsal, and cavernosal arteries. The paired cavernosal arteries penetrate the tunica albuginea, and terminate in multiple twisted branches called helicine arterioles that supply the lacunar spaces. Venous return from the penis occurs via the deep and superficial dorsal veins of the penis. Subtunical venules located between the erectile tissue and the tunica albuginea drain the lacunar spaces. Superficial dorsal veins communi-cate with the external pudendal vein and/or the saphenous vein to drain the skin and prepuce of the penis. Penile erection occurs in response to sensory stimuli, fantasy, or genital stimulation. Sympathetic pregangli-onic nerve fibers to the penis arise from neurons in the T12-L2 spinal cord segments, while parasympathetic input to the penis arises in the S2-S4 segments. Sympathetic impulses travel via the hypogastric nerve, and parasympathetic impulses travel via the pelvic nerve. The pelvic plexus serves as the peripheral integration center for autonomic input to the penis. The pelvic plexus branches into the cavernous nerves that traverse the posterolateral aspect of the prostate and continue on both sides of the urethra as the cavernosal nerves. In the flaccid state, there is tonic contraction of the arterial and corporal smooth muscles medi-ated by $\alpha$–2 adrenergic receptors. With erotic stimulation, there is a decrease in sympathetic impulses and an increase in parasympathetic activity. Parasympathetic stimulation activates cholinergic receptors, stimulating endothelial cells to produce a nonadrenergic, noncholinergic transmitter—nitric oxide (NO). NO relaxes trabecular smooth muscle, and is considered the major neurotransmitter controlling relaxation of penile smooth muscle. Other entities have been implicated in the control of erection, including prostaglandins $E_1$ (PGE$_1$) and $E_2$ (PGE$_2$) and vasoactive peptide (VP). Tonic sympathetic stimulation constricts the trabecular smooth muscle and helicine arterioles keeping the penis flaccid. During flaccidity, blood pressure in the cavernosal lacunae is similar to venous pressure. With sexual stimulation, sympathetic tone decreases and there is parasympathetic-mediated relaxation of arteriolar and trabecular smooth muscle. Penile arterial resistance decreases resulting in increased blood flow into the corpora cavernosa. The increase in blood volume expands the lacunar spaces, and compresses the subtunical venules between the expanding corpora cavernosa and the unyielding tunica albuginea. This results in reduction of venous outflow and trapping of blood within the penis. Penile rigidity develops as intracavernosal pressure rises to mean arterial pressure. Detumescence typically occurs after orgasm. During detumescence, there is a decrease in the arterial flow into the penis, decrease in intracavernosal pressure, increased venous drainage, and restoration of sympathetic nerve impulses returning the penis to the flaccid state (Lue 2000).

### E. Treatment Approaches

1. Diagnostic work-up

   a. Part of any diagnostic evaluation is a thorough history and physical exam including psychosocial assessment and sexual history. Patients presenting with complaints of ED may have an undiagnosed medical condition as coronary artery disease. Often, treatment of the underlying medical condition will relieve the symptoms of ED. In addition, medication usage as well as recreation drug use should be reviewed and ruled out as a source of ED.

   b. Laboratory exams are indicated to rule out general medical conditions or endocrine sources. These labs include a basic chemistry panel with random blood sugar, complete blood count, free and bound testosterone, lutenizing hormone, and prolactin levels. Liver function tests are also useful to detect any hepatic impairment and will serve as a baseline measure if papaverine cavernosal injections are used to treat ED. In addition a screening prostate-specific antigen (PSA) should be done if routine screening has not been initiated or maintained.

c. Diagnostic modalities used to assess ED include color duplex Doppler ultrasonography with and without pharmacostimulation, dynamic infusion cavernosography/cavernosometry, and pelvic angiography, which are useful in evaluating vascular insufficiency or veno-occlusive defect. To differentiate between psychosocial and biological etiologies, nocturnal penile tumescence monitoring is useful. Less commonly used tests include penile/brachial pressure index, nuclear washout radiography, and magnetic resonance angiography.

2. **Biological treatments**

   a. Pharmacotherapy

      1) Oral medications play a major role in the treatment of ED. Since the introduction of the PDE–5 inhibitor sildenafil (Viagra®), there have been two additions to this class of drugs: vardenafil HCL (Levitra®) and tadalafil (Cialis®). These drugs essentially have become the first line agents in the treatment of ED and essentially share the same mechanism of action with some variance in their half lives and side effect profile. These medications are contraindicated in patients taking nitrates and should be used judiciously in patients with cardiovascular disease (Lue 2003). The side effects include nasal congestion, headache, flushing, dyspepsia, and visual changes. With respect to tadalafil, there has been reported myalgia and back pain. More details about oral medications are presented in Chapter 2 on the Biopsychosocial Evaluation and Treatment of Sexual Disorders.

         a) Recommended starting dosage of sildenafil is 50mg, which may be increased to a maximum recommended dose of 100mg or decreased to 25mg never exceeding max dosing frequency of once per day. Concurrent use of alpha–1 blockers for hypertension or benign prostatic hypertrophy BPH is also cautioned in dosages greater than 25mg. Sildenafil must be taken at least four hours apart from an alpha–1 blocker secondary to risk of severe hypotension. In addition, sildenafil may be taken anywhere between 30 minutes to 4 hours prior to sexual activity, but is recommended to be taken 1 hour before sexual activity on an empty stomach.

b)  Vardenafil is supplied in 2.5 mg, 5 mg, 10 mg, and 20 mg tablets. The recommended starting dose is 10 mg, which can be increased to 20 mg or decreased not to exceed once a day dosing. Recommendations for patients with moderate hepatic impairment (Child-Pugh B) include a starting dose of 5 mg not to exceed a maximal dose of 10 mg. Vardenafil is contraindicated in patients using alpha–1 inhibitors and no dose adjustment is required in patients regardless of degree of renal insufficiency although it has not been studied in patients on renal dialysis. Sildenafil and vardenafil have a similar half-life ranging 4–6 hours.

c)  Tadalafil has the longest reported half-life shown to improve erectile function for up to 36 hours when compared to placebo thus potentially prolonging the side effect profile for that entire period. Recommend starting dosage is 10mg which may be increased to a maximal dose of 20 mg or decreased to 5 mg as needed, never to exceed a dose frequency of once a day. Tadalafil is supplied in 5 mg, 10 mg, and 20 mg preparations. Use of tadalafil with alpha–1 blockers is contraindicated except with tamsulosin (Flomax®) 0.4mg each day only. In patients with mild or moderate hepatic impairment should not exceed a maximal dose of 10 mg while in patients with severe hepatic dysfunction (Child-Pugh Class C) the use of tadalafil is not recommended. In patients with moderate renal insufficiency (creatinine clearance 31–50 mL/min) recommended starting and maximal doses are 5 mg once daily and 10 mg once every 48 hours respectively. For patients with severe renal insufficiency (creatinine clearance <30 mL/min) on hemodialysis, the maximal recommended dose is 5 mg.

d)  There are no head-to-head trials comparing the three PDE–5 inhibitors. Gresser and Gleiter (2002) reviewed a significant number of studies on the three medications. They concluded that efficacy is approximately 70% with the three medications with similar side effect profile. Vasodilatation leading to headaches, nasal congestion, and flushing, are common but rarely cause subjects to drop out of clinical trials (2–3%). Two side effects seem to stand out: blue vision (due to PDE–6 inhibition in the retina) is seen only with Viagra (<0.5%) and muscle aches are seen only with Cialis (5%). Nitrates are contraindicated with all three. The long half-life of tadalafil (16–18 hours) was noted to extend to its effects to a whole weekend earning it its nicknames 'weekender' or 'weekend pill'.

2) Another oral agent yohimbine, which has not shown to be effective for ED, however, it does appear effective in patients with inorganic etiologies (Ernst et al. 1998). Yohimbine is typically dosed at 5.4 mg orally three times a day. Androgen supplementation may be warranted in-patients with hypogonadal states and decreased libido. Other agents include phentolamine, apomorphine, and the combination of trazadone and yohimbine, which have shown to improve symptoms of ED, but are not currently FDA approved for this treatment.

3) Apomorphine: 2–3mg 20–30 minutes PO or SL before intercourse has been clinically proven to start acting within 15–30 minutes—two to three times faster than Viagra. Recent studies have shown that following the administration of sublingual apomorphine 34% of erections were reached within 10 minutes and 71% within 20 minutes. Side effects: The most commonly found ones are headache, dizziness and nausea—with dizziness occurring in approximately 4% of patients, and nausea and headache occurring in approximately 7% of patients. Nausea is usually mild to moderate, and tends to dissipate with prolonged use of the drug. Other adverse side effects include: infection; pain; flushing; taste disorder; sweating; yawning; rhinitus; pharyngitis, somno-

lence, increased cough. Currently, apomorphine is not FDA approved for the treatment of ED.

4) Alprostadil (prostaglandin $E_1$) cream: 1,700 patients with mild to severe ED are enrolled in the two Phase 3 studies of Alprox-TD Cream. The pre-measured dose is applied locally to the tip of the penis with the onset of activity reported at 10–15 minutes patients reported improvement in their erections of 83 percent, 76 percent and 59 percent in the High, Medium and Low dose groups, respectively, versus 26 percent in the placebo group. Side effects were primarily localized at the site of application and were mild to moderate in nature. The overall discontinuance rate due to side effects was 3%.

5) Transurethral alprostadil (MUSE®) is a second line therapy that has shown effectiveness, but is associated with moderate to severe penile pain, moderate response rates, and inconsistent efficacy (Porst 1997). MUSE® has been shown to be effective in 30% of men who try it with onset of action occurring within 10–15 minutes of application lasting approximately 30–60 minutes. These pellets are prepared in 125, 250, and 500 microgram preparations and can used up to two times in a 24 hour period, not to be given immediately following resolution of the first erections.

6) Intracavernosal therapy is highly effective in both psychosocial and neurogenic ED; however, the response rate is less in patients with arterial insufficiency. It is a second line agent and can be administered as a single agent using papaverine (a phosphodiesterase inhibitor) or alprostadil. Tri-mix using these two agents in combination with phentolamine, an alpha-adrenergic receptor antagonist, is very effective with response rates as high as 90% (Bennett et al. 1991). First dose should be administered under observation of a physician to ensure proper technique by the patient as well as ensure adequate dosing. Dosages can be titrated on an individual basis. Typical dosages for injectable papaverine and alprostadil are 30 to 60 mg and 1.25 to 60 micrograms (mcg) respectively. The dosage of phentolamine ranges from 0.5 to

1 mg. Cavernosal injections should be avoided in patients with bleeding tendencies or history of sickle cell disease. Disadvantages of intracavernosal injections include risk of priapism, corporeal fibrosis, pain at the injection site, and loss of spontaneity.

7) Vacuum constriction devices are also available and are effective as a second line therapy for the treatment of ED. It has no systemic side effects, but maybe associated with localized symptoms of numbness and petechiae. Vacuum devices typically consist of three main components including a plastic cylinder, pump (manual versus battery operated) to create vacuum pressure, and tension rings used to constrict the base of the penis in order to maintain the erection. These devices also cause trapped ejaculation and are considered cumbersome with loss of spontaneity.

b. Surgical treatments

1) Developed in the early 1970s, penile prosthesis is a highly effective treatment modality for patients that have failed medical treatment. The two primary types are semi rigid and inflatable devices. These devices have been associated with infection and some require replacement after 5–10 years. Semi rigid malleable (positioning) rods are typically reserved for patients with poor manual dexterity who would be unable to self-inflate the device or in patients with previous history of significant abdominal/pelvic surgery where a reservoir could not be placed for three piece inflatable device. This latter problem maybe obviated with the use of a two piece inflatable device. In addition, medical co-pays may influence a patient's decision against the more expensive inflatable devices. The malleable rods are typically made of a silicone outer coating with interlocking plastic joints connected by a stainless steel core enabling the patient to place the penis in an erect or flaccid position. A three-piece inflatable device includes two inflatable cylinders, which are inserted into each corpus cavernosum and connected to a reservoir containing saline solution via manual pump, which is typically placed in

the scrotum. The reservoir is typically placed in the extra-peritoneal space in the pelvis. Penile prosthetic surgery is completed on an outpatient basis or "23 hour stay" protocol. Patients are to refrain from using the devices for approximately 4–6 weeks post-operatively to ensure proper healing and to ensure the reservoir space develops to reduce the incidence of auto-inflation secondary to decreased capacitance in this extraperitoneal space.

2) Arterial revascularization procedures have poor results in older patients and typically are more efficacious in younger men with congenital or traumatic ED. Venous ligation is not effective in the treatment of ED.

### 3. Psychosocial treatments

This noninvasive partner involved treatment is considered a first line treatment for psychosocial or combined ED. In addition, it maybe used in combination with other treatments. Sex Therapy: Sensate Focus is a series of specific exercises for couples that encourages each partner to take turns paying increased attention to their own senses. These exercises were originally developed by Masters and Johnson to assist couples experiencing sexual problems, but can be used for variety and to heighten personal awareness with any couple. When used in the treatment setting, sensate focus is done in several stages over the course of therapy.

### 4. Communication and education

Discussing the erectile disorder and its physiology helps men and their partners understand and accurately estimate the issues, and reassures them of the availability of treatment interventions and favorable prognosis. Education often provides immediate relief and helps prepare the couple for the treatment course.

### F. Prognosis

The management of ED was revolutionized by two key developments. The first took place in the early 1970s with the advent of the penile prosthesis. This new treatment modality changed the focus from inorganic causes of ED to biologic etiologies. The second turning point occurred with the introduction of the type 5 phosphodiesterase (PDE–5) inhibitors in the late 1990s.

With modern pharmacological, surgical, and behavioral treatments, most ED patients can be cured with single or multiple modality therapy. With respect to pharmacological treatments there is a risk of developing of drug resistance secondary to worsening medical conditions as well as the theoretical development of drug tolerance. Also when pharmacological failure occurs, patient's drug administration should be reviewed. Current literature suggests that patients' responses to PDE–5 inhibitors are improved when a urologist versus a general practitioner provides instructions (Atiemo et al. 2003). Some ED patients requiring pharmacological assistance have shown an increased rate of spontaneous erections at times not requiring further pharmacotherapy. This phenomenon appears more common in the post-operative patients. In addition, some patients, depending on the etiology will require lifelong treatment for the management of ED.

## III. Female Sexual Arousal Disorder

### A. Definition and Phenomenology

Female sexual arousal disorder (FSAD) is defined by the DSM-IV-TR (APA 2000) as the persistent or recurrent inability to attain or maintain an adequate lubrication-swelling response of sexual excitement until completion of sexual activity resulting in marked distress or interpersonal difficulty. In normal arousal responses, pelvic vasocongestion occurs with associated vaginal lubrication as well as the enlargement and swelling of the external genitalia. Sexual arousal disorder must cause marked distress or interpersonal difficulties and must be excluded from the effects of a substance or general medical condition.

Women with FSAD may experience pain or discomfort with intercourse due to decreased lubrication and swelling. Some patients may note diminished capacity for vaginal or clitoral sensation as well as diminished vaginal or clitoral orgasm. Various forms of FSAD include lifelong versus acquired type as well as generalized versus situational type. The etiology of the dysfunction should also be differentiated between psychological factors versus combined factors. Five subtypes of FSAD have been described and include: generalized arousal disor-

---

**TABLE 2**

**Diagnostic Criteria for 302.72 Female Sexual Arousal Disorder**

A. Persistent or recurrent inability to attain, or to maintain until completion of the sexual activity, an adequate lubrication-swelling response of sexual excitement.

B. The disturbance causes marked distress or interpersonal difficulty.

C. The Male Erectile Disorder is not better accounted for by another Axis I disorder (other than a Sexual Dysfunction) and is not due exclusively to the direct physiological effects of a substance (e.g., a drug of abuse, a medication) or a general medical condition.

Specify type:   Lifelong Type

Acquired Type

Specify type:   Generalized Type

Situational Type

Specify:   Due to Psychological Factors

Due to Combined Factors

Reprinted with permission from the Diagnostic and Statistical Manual of Mental Disorders, Fourth Edition, Text Revision. Copyright 2000 American Psychiatric Association

---

der, genital arousal disorder, missed arousal disorder, dysphoric arousal disorder, and anhedonic arousal disorder (Basson et al. 2003).

More emphasis is put on this disorder in the context of Chapter 10 on Women's Sexual Health.

## B. Epidemiology

Sexual dysfunction in general affects 43% of women (Laumann et al. 1999). The prevalence of FSAD is estimated to be 20% (Rosen 2000).

## C. Etiology

Analogous to male ED, women may experience FSAD secondary to physiologic as well as psychosocial sources.

### 1. Biological factors

a. Risk factors for sexual arousal disorder in women include age of the patient, level of education, and physical health (Goldstein 2000). Genetic reasons for FSAD are largely unknown.

b. Substance-induced FSAD: alcohol, illicit drugs, prescription and over the counter medications, dietary supplements and herbs in addition to toxins could cause FSAD. An extensive discussion of substances affecting sexual functioning is presented in Chapter 3 on Substance-induced Sexual Dysfunction.

c. Medical factors:

1) Central and peripheral neuropathies. Neuropathies may stem from spinal cord injury as well as diabetic induced neuropathy.

2) Vascular problems including atherosclerosis, hyperlipidemia, hypertension, and diabetes may lead to microvascular disease and subsequent arterial insufficiency.

3) Trauma, irradiation or previous pelvic surgery may lead to both peripheral nerve injury and arterial insufficiency.

4) Endocrinal: Hormonal imbalances such as low testosterone, low estrogen, increased prolactin could all affect sexual arousal. Postmenopausal and lactating women report difficulties with sexual arousal.

## 2. Psychosocial factors

a. Psychiatric Disorders: Mood Disorders especially depression, and Anxiety Disorders.

b. Stressors: traumas, losses, and conflicts in addition to financial, vocational, and residential factors. History of sexual abuse is a well-recognized cause of FSAD.

c. Relational issues such as relationship conflicts, feeling pressured or forced, anger, lack of trust, lack of attractiveness to the partner, and lack of adequacy of sexual stimulation.

## D. Pathophysiology

FSAD may be caused by psychosocial and or biologic factors. With normal sexual arousal there is increased pelvic vasocongestion leading to engorgement of the vagina, and external genitalia. As clitoral erection and vaginal length and luminal diameter increases, transudation of plasma occurs allowing flow onto the vaginal surface. Any disruption of this path can lead to FSAD. Regarding pelvic irradiation, renewing epithelial cells of the vagina are altered, loosing their transudative and elastic properties stunting the lubrication-swelling response. Inadequate hormonal milieu during menopause or after surgical castration also leads to mucosal changes and diminished sexual arousal response. As in men, certain medical conditions as mentioned above have been associated with FSAD.

### E. Treatment Approaches

1. Diagnostic work-up

   a. A thorough history and physical is essential in evaluating patients with sexual dysfunction. Sexual history should take into account the focus, intensity, and duration of sexual activity as well as the adequacy of sexual stimulation.

   b. Laboratory examination will help to evaluate any general medical conditions. Theses studies include chemistry and hormonal panel including a random blood sugar, complete blood count and liver function tests, which will rule out any hepatic impairment and also serve as a baseline levels if hormonal replacement is instituted. The hormonal panel should include estradiol levels, free and bound testosterone, follicle stimulating hormone (FSH), and lutenizing hormone (LH).

   c. Duplex Doppler sonography, photoplethysmography, or measurement of vaginal and labial oxygen tensions may be used in measuring genital blood flow. Recordings at baseline and after sexual stimulation are helpful in determining pathologic changes. Other available diagnostic tools to evaluate neuropathic changes include measurement of bulbocavernosus reflex and pudendal evoked potentials, genital sympathetic skin response, warm, cold, vibratory perception thresholds, and pressure/touch sensitivity of the external genitalia.

2. Biological treatments:

   a. Treatment of the underlying medical conditions and removal or substitutions of substances interfering with arousal are of prime importance. More details about the treatment strategies of substance-induced sexual disorders are provided in Chapter 2 on Biopsychosocial Evaluation and Treatment of Sexual Disorder.

b. Primary therapy for FSAD at this time is hormone replacement therapy (HRT). Various replacement modalities exist while the use of local or topical agents help relieve vaginal symptoms of dryness and burning, as well as urinary urgency and frequency. Topical estrogen has also been shown to increase clitoral sensitivity and decrease pain/burning during intercourse. Estrogen cream does not relieve sexual complaints other that local vaginal pain or dryness. Patients should be advised of the risks associated with HRT including long-term risk of coronary heart disease, stroke, invasive breast cancer, and pulmonary embolism (Rossouw et al. 2002).

c. Testosterone in the form of methyltestosterone used in combination with estrogen (Estratest®/EstratestHS®) has also been used to treat FSAD. This FDA approved treatment is typically reserved for postmenopausal women to help treat patients with decreased vaginal lubrication and those with inhibited desire. Patients should be counseled on risks of possible hair growth and deepening voice.

d. PDE-5 inhibitor, sildenafil, has been evaluated in both pre and post-menopausal women. In a recent study by Caruso et al. (2003), there was a statistically significant improvement over placebo with respect to sexual arousal, orgasm, and enjoyment in young asymptomatic cohort of premenopausal women. In another study reviewed by Baty (2001) looking at young premenoupausal women with FSAD, sildenafil significantly increased sexual arousal scores and frequency of orgasm compared to placebo. Sildenafil has also shown some benefit in postmenopausal women with FSAD without concomitant hypoactive sexual desire disorder (Berman et al. 2003). Side effects among female subjects include headache, flushing, visual disturbances, rhinitis and nausea.

e. Sildenafil, yohimbine, L-Arginine, phentolamine, topical alprostadil (prostaglandin $E_1$), apomorphine, and selective serotonin re-uptake inhibitors (SSRI) are still considered investigational in the management of female sexual disorders at this time.

f. Clitoral vacuum device such as the Eros Clitoral Therapy Device (EROS-CTD) is safe and effective in improving symptoms of FSAD, including increased sensation, improved vaginal lubrication, and enhanced ability to orgasm (Wilson et al. 2001).

g. A blend of natural ingredients (Borage seed oil, Evening primrose oil, Angelica root extract, and Coleus extract) named Zestra was shown to ameliorate FSAD even when caused by SSRIs when topically applied (Ferguson et al. 2003).

## 3. Psychosocial treatments

This is a first line treatment for inorganic etiologies of FSAD and should involve partner participation although there are no efficacy reports regarding this modality.

a. Treatment of underlying psychiatric disorders is of prime importance.

b. Sex therapy provides a practical approach to arousal problems by shifting focus from lubrication and penetration to mutual pleasurable touch during sensate focus exercises. Working the way gradually back to genital contact is done when the couple had mastered communication and pleasure techniques. Sex Therapy is described in full details in Chapter 2 on the Biopsychosocial Evaluation and Treatment of Sexual Disorder.

c. Couple therapy provides a venue to work through communication and commitment problems.

b. Individual psychotherapy is highly indicated in cases of sexual trauma, significant interpersonal problems and in women with lifelong, and generalized arousal disorders.

## 4. Communication and education

Discussing the female sexual arousal disorder and its physiology helps women and their partners understand and accurately estimate the issues, and reassures them of the availability of treatment interventions and favorable prognosis. Education often provides immediate relief and helps prepare the couple for the treatment course.

**F. Prognosis**

The understanding of FSAD is still in its infancy awaiting further research in biologic etiologies and pharmacological treatments. With better understanding, FSAD may be treated efficiently with single or combined modalities.

## IV. Conclusion and Future Directions

The incidence of ED and FSAD increases with age and are typically due to combined factors. With the introduction of PDE–5 inhibitors, we have witnessed an increased awareness to the subject of sexual dysfunction now being managed by a variety of medical services. As previously mentioned, most forms of ED and FSAD are treatable and may require single or combined treatment modalities. Pharmacological studies comparing the various PDE–5 inhibitors would aid in developing a specific protocol for patient and drug selection and administration. The potential use of gene therapy/transfer (locally administered) for the treatment of bladder and erectile dysfunction has been reviewed (Christ 2004). With FSAD, further studies evaluating the effects of pelvic surgery or irradiation are needed to better understand and predict post procedural outcomes in women. Other areas of future direction may focus on neuromodulation with an implantable device to alleviate the symptoms of FSAD.

## *References*

Atiemo HO, Szostak MJ, Sklar GN: Salvage of sildenafil failures referred from primary care physicians. J Urol 170(6 Pt 1):2356–2358, 2003

Basson R, Leiblum S, Brotto L, et al.: Definitions of women's sexual dysfunction reconsidered: advocating expansion and revision. J Psychosom Obstet Gynaecol 24(4):221–229, 2003

Baty PJ: Is sildenafil (Viagra) an efficacious treatment for sexual arousal disorder in premenopausal women? J Fam Pract 50(11):921 2001

Bennett AH, Carpenter AJ, Barada JH: An improved vasoactive drug combination for a pharmacological erection program. J Urol 146:1564–1565, 1991

Berman JR, Berman LA, Toler SM, et al.: Safety and efficacy of sildenafil citrate for the treatment of female sexual arousal disorder: a double-blind, placebo controlled study. J Urol 170(6):2333–2338, 2003

Berman JR, Shuker JM, Goldstein I: Female sexual dysfunction. In Carson C, Kirby R, Goldstein I (editors): Textbook of erectile dysfunction. Isis Medical Media Ltd, Oxford, UK:627–638, 1999

Caruso S, Intlisano G, Farina M, et al.: The function of sildenafil on female sexual pathways: a double-blind, cross-over, placebo-controlled study. Eur J Obstet Gynecol Reprod Biol 110:01–206, 2003

Christ GJ: Gene therapy treatments for erectile and bladder dysfunction. Current Urology Reports 5(1):52–60, 2004

Ernst E, Pittler MH: Yohimbine for erectile dysfunction: a systematic review and meta-analysis of randomized clinical trials. J Urol 159(2):433–436, 1998

Feldman HA, Goldstein I, Hatzichristou DG, et al.: Impotence and its medical and psychosocial correlates: results of the Massachusetts male aging study. J Urol 151(1):54–61, 1994

Ferguson DM, Singh GS, Steidle CP, et al.: Randomized, Placebo-Controlled, Double Blind, Crossover Design Trial of the Efficacy and Safety of Zestra for Women in Women With and Without Female Sexual Arousal Disorder. Journal of Sex & Marital Therapy 29 (1) Supp. 1: 33–44, 2003

Fischer ME, Vitek ME, Hedeker D, et al.: A twin study of erectile dysfunction. Archives of Internal Medicine 164(2):165–8, 2004

Goldstein I: Female sexual arousal disorder: new insights. Int J Impot Res 12 Suppl 4:S152-S157, 2000

Gresser U, Gleiter CH: Erectile dysfunction: Comparison of efficacy and side effects of the PDE–5 inhibitors sildenafil, vardenafil and tadalafil. European Journal of Medical Research, 7(10): 435–446, 2002

Kirby RS: Basic assessment of the patient with erectile dysfunction. In Carson C, Kirby R, Goldstein I (editors): Textbook of erectile dysfunction. Oxford, UK: Isis Medical Media Ltd, 195–205, 1999

Laumann EO, Paik AM, Rosen RC: Sexual dysfunction in the United States: prevalence and predictors. JAMA 281(6):537–544, 1999

Lue TF: Erectile dysfunction. NEJM 342:1802–1813, 2000

Marthol H, Hilz MJ: Female sexual dysfunction: a systematic overview of classification, pathophysiology, diagnosis and treatment. Fortschr Neurol Psychiatr 72(3):121–135, 2004

Porst H: Transurethral alprostadil with MUSE (medicated urethral system for erection) vs intracavernous alprostadil—a comparative study in 103 patients with erectile dysfunction. Int J Impot Res 9:187–192, 1997

Rosen RC: Prevalence and risk factors of sexual dysfunction in men and women. Current Psychiatry Reports 2(3):189–95, 2000

Rossouw JE, Anderson GL, Prentice RL, et al: Risks and benefits of estrogen plus progestin in healthy postmenopausal women: principal results from the women's health initiative randomized controlled trial. JAMA 288(3):321–333, 2002

Seftel AD: Erectile Disorder in the elderly: epidemiology, etiology and approaches to treatment. J Urol 169(6):1999–2007, 2003

Wilson SK, Delk JR, Billups KL: Treating symptoms of female sexual arousal disorder with the Eros-Clitoral Therapy Device. J Gend Specif Med 4(2):54–58, 2001

# 7

# Orgasmic Disorders

Waguih William IsHak, M.D.
Laura Berman, Ph.D.
Kerrie Grow McLean, Psy.D.

## I. Introduction

Orgasmic disorders according to the DSM-IV-TR (APA 2000) include three categories of disorders: Premature Ejaculation, Female Orgasmic Disorder and Male Orgasmic Disorder. Each disorder is defined below.

### Premature Ejaculation

Persistent or recurrent ejaculation with minimal sexual stimulation or before, on, or shortly after penetration and before the person wishes it, resulting in marked distress or interpersonal difficulty. The clinician must take into account factors that affect duration of the excitement phase, such as age, novelty of the sexual partner or situation, and frequency of sexual activity.

### Female Orgasmic Disorder

Persistent or recurrent delay in, or absence of, orgasm in a female following a normal sexual excitement phase, resulting in marked distress or interpersonal difficulty while it is not better accounted for by another Axis I disorder (apart from other sexual disorders). The diagnosis of Female Orgasmic Disorder should be based on the clinician's judgment that the woman's orgasmic capacity is less than would be reasonable for her age, sexual experience, and the adequacy of sexual stimulation she receives.

### Male Orgasmic Disorder

Persistent or recurrent delay in, or absence of, orgasm following a normal sexual excitement phase during sexual activity, resulting in marked distress or interpersonal difficulty while it is not better accounted for by another Axis I disorder (apart from other sexual disorders). The diagnosis of Male Orgasmic Disorder should be based on the clinician's judgment taking into account the person's age, adequacy of stimulation in focus, intensity, and duration.

### Other Orgasm Disorders

These include Retrograde Ejaculation in Men, and Orgasmic Cephalgia (headache) in women.

## II. Premature Ejaculation (PE)

### A. Definition and Phenomenology

As defined below, PE is the persistent or recurrent ejaculation with minimal sexual stimulation or before, on, or shortly after penetration and before the person wishes it, resulting in marked distress or interpersonal difficulty. PE is sometimes referred to as Rapid Ejaculation.

The average ejaculatory latency (self-reported in a community survey or reported in the laboratory) is around a mean of 7.9 minutes (Grenier et al. 2001, and Kameya et al. 1997). The normal physical response for women to build to orgasm is about 12 to 14 minutes after coitus occurs. PE definition has been one of the barriers to getting

**TABLE 1**
**DSM-IV Diagnostic Criteria for 302.75 Premature Ejaculation**

A. Persistent or recurrent ejaculation with minimal sexual stimulation before, on, or shortly after penetration and before the person wishes it. The clinician must take into account factors that affect duration of the excitement phase, such as age, novelty of the sexual partner or situation, and recent frequency of sexual activity.

B. The disturbance causes marked distress or interpersonal difficulty.

C. The premature ejaculation is not due exclusively to the direct effects of a substance (e.g., withdrawal from opioids).

| | |
|---|---|
| Specify type: | Lifelong Type |
| | Acquired Type |
| Specify type: | Generalized Type |
| | Situational Type |
| Specify: | Due to Psychological Factors |
| | Due to Combined Factors |

Reprinted with permission from the Diagnostic and Statistical Manual of Mental Disorders, Fourth Edition, Text Revision. Copyright 2000 American Psychiatric Association

consistency among studies. However, a large number of studies have attributed the difficulty of PE definition to self-identification. The primary symptom is persistent or recurrent episodes of premature ejaculation during sex. Another historical, clinical definition is when ejaculation occurs less than two minutes of penetration during more than fifty percent of intercourse experiences for at least six months duration. Secondary symptoms may include: feelings of guilt, inadequacy, or self-doubt, and new or increased interpersonal problems with a sexual partner. Types of PE include Lifelong Type/Acquired Type, Generalized Type/Situational Type and Due to Psychological Factors or Due to Combined Factors.

## B. Epidemiology

In more recent sexual behavior surveys in the United States, almost one-third of men said they had recurring problems with ejaculating prematurely, making it the most common sexual disorder in men. Rates seem to be higher in black men (34%), and lower in Hispanic men

(27%) as compared to White men (29%). The rates were also higher in less educated men (35% in high school graduates and 38% in less than high school education) compared to some college educated or college graduates (26% and 27% respectively), but do not appear to change with age or marital status (Laumann et al. 1999).

## C. Etiology

### 1. Biological factors:

a. General: Psychopharmacological treatment studies, animal research data and stopwatch assessments in men with lifelong PE indicate that the disorder is related to diminished serotonergic neurotransmission, 5-HT2c or 5-HT1A receptor disturbances and likely influenced by hereditary factors (Waldinger 2002 and 2004). Kameya, Deguchi, and Yokota (1997) have demonstrated individual differences in ejaculatory latency even given the same sexual stimulation under similar conditions. Greater penile sensitivity and a shorter bulbocavernosus reflex nerve response latency have both been linked to some cases of primary PE (Metz et al., 1997; Rowland & Slob, 1997). Men who reported having more frequent intercourse also reported longer ejaculatory latencies, greater ejaculatory control, less concern over ejaculating too soon, greater satisfaction with the ability to select the moment of ejaculation, and a lower percentage of intercourse occasions when they ejaculated too quickly, and were less likely to identify themselves as having a problem with PE (Grenier et al. 2001). These findings are consistent with Gospodinoff (1989) and Spiess et al. (1984) who reported that greater periods of sexual abstinence correlated positively with shorter ejaculatory latencies.

b. Infections: Chronic prostatitis and urethritis have been implicated in PE. Italian researchers massaged the prostates of men with premature ejaculation, examined their semen, and found an infection in 56 percent and specific bacteria grew in 47 percent. The control group had a much lower incidence of infection (Screponi et al. 2001).

   c. Arteriosclerosis and cardiovascular disease have been identified as contributing to PE.

   d. Benign prostatic hyperplasia and urinary incontinence have been implicated in many cases of PE.

   e. Drugs such as over the counter cold pills and cigarette smoking were identified as contributing to PE. Withdrawal from opiates has been associated with PE (APA 2000).

   f. Other factors include Diabetes Mellitus, pelvic and spinal cord injuries, polyneuritis, and polycythemia.

   g. Animal studies showed that mice lacking the gene for endothelial nitric oxide synthase develop a PE-like condition while mice lacking the gene for heme oxygenase–2 exhibit delayed ejaculation (Abdel-Hamid 2004).

2. **Psychosocial factors:**

   a. Past experiences: The classical view first advanced by Masters and Johnson (1970) is that men who have initial intercourse experiences that are rushed, either because their first partner(s) wished intercourse to end quickly or because there was a danger of being caught or discovered while having intercourse, become conditioned to ejaculate rapidly. Age, number of sexual partners, feeling rushed during early intercourse experiences, and experiencing negative affect during these early experiences found little support in studies reported by Grenier et al. (1997, 2001) and Laumann et al. (1999).

   b. Anxiety: Premature ejaculation often occurs during first experiences with sex, and is most commonly attributed to anxiety. Longer-term performance anxiety also contributes to premature ejaculation. PE may also be caused or aggravated by psychological factors such as guilt (e.g., premarital or extramarital sex) fear (associated with concerns regarding potential pregnancy, sexually transmitted diseases, or getting caught or discovered); and performance anxiety (especially in the inexperienced partner or with partners new to each other)

   c. Relational: Interpersonal issues affecting the couple could cause PE.

d) Psychiatric disorders (see Appendix 3): Premature ejaculation was the most common sexual dysfunction in male patients with social phobia, occurring in nearly half of those patients (Figueira et al. 2001).

## D. Pathophysiology

The physiology of ejaculation includes an impulse, which is visual, physical or both, travels to the spinal cord and then to the brain where the autonomic nervous system stimulates the sympathetic nerves. This sacral-spinal reflex mediated by the pudendal nerve results in contraction of the male accessory sexual organs including the vas deferens, the tube that carries sperm from the testicles to the prostate. The prostate itself generates part of the fluid that comprises the ejaculate as it passes on its way. There is even a small contribution from the bulbourethral glands, also known as Cowpers gland, located just before the beginning of the penis. An ejaculation actually occurs when this fluid is propelled out of the penis by a contraction of the bulbocavernosus and the levator ani muscles, which comprise part of the pelvic floor leading to emission of sperm with the accessory gland fluid into the urethra, simultaneous closure of the urethral sphincters, and forceful ejaculation of semen through the urethra. Emission and closure of the bladder neck are primarily alpha-adrenergically mediated thoracolumbar sympathetic reflex events with supraspinal modulation. This modulation involves serotonergic and noradrenergic activities. Atamac et al. found that serum leptin (an adipocyte hormone involved in appetite suppression) levels were high in patients with premature ejaculation and lowered after 8 weeks of citalopram treatment (Atamac et al. 2003). Although there is no direct evidence of an association involving brain pathways related to sexual behavior, there is an interaction between leptinergic and serotonergic systems.

## E. Treatment Approaches

1. Diagnostic work-up:

   a. Interview the couple in depth to gather more specific information about PE.

   b. Medical work-up should include excluding general medical problems, urinary tract infections, Prostatitis, and identification of any substance related effects. More specialized laboratory testing might be indicated such as ejaculatory latency.

2. **Biological and physical treatments:**

   a. General: Medical treatment for PE includes the treatment of primary medical conditions and the identification and cessation of use of substances responsible for premature ejaculation. For many years behavioral therapy was the only treatment available and accepted: the start-stop method (Semans 1956) and the squeeze method (Masters & Johnson 1970). In recent years a number of studies have been carried out to test the efficacy of psychopharmacological drugs, more specifically anti-depressants (Crenshaw & Goldberg 1996; Riley, Peet, & Wilson 1993; Rowland, Cooper, & Slob 1998; Rowland & Slob 1997; Waldinger 1997). Most of the drugs (e.g., clomipramine and paroxetine) appeared to be fairly effective in postponing ejaculation (Rowland et al., 1998), both when taken on a daily basis (Waldinger, Hengeveld, Zwinderman, & Olivier 1998) and when taken as needed, about 1 to 24 hrs before anticipated sexual activity (Haensel, Rowland, Kallan, & Slob 1997; Strassberg, de Gouveia Brazao, Rowland, Tan, & Slob 1999). An alternative type of treatment is the local application of an anesthetic ointment to the penis.

   b. Physical:

      1) Condoms are an effective means of reducing the amount of stimulation experienced during sex.

      2) Some therapists advise young men to masturbate (or have their partner stimulate them rapidly to climax) 1–2 hours before sexual relations are planned. The interval for achieving a second climax often includes a much longer latency period, and the male can usually exert better control in this setting. In an older man, such a strategy may be less effective because the older man may have difficulty achieving a second erection after his first rapid sexual release. If this occurs, it can damage his confidence and may result in secondary impotence.

      3) Sexual positions: trying different sexual positions that may allow greater control over the muscles that cause ejaculation.

The woman (or partner) on top is one of the well-known positions to ameliorate PE.

c. Medications:

1) Selective Serotonin reuptake inhibitors (SSRIs): No drug is approved by the FDA for the treatment of PE. However, numerous studies have shown that SSRIs and drugs with SSRI-like side effects are safe and effective to treat this condition, and many physicians use these agents for this purpose. Many of these agents have been found to have, as a side effect, a tendency to cause both male and female patients to experience a significant delay in reaching orgasm. Mechanism of action is linked to their inhibition of neuronal uptake of serotonin in the CNS. In men with pre-mature ejaculation 20 mg of fluoxetine 6–12 hours before intercourse or 20 mg on daily basis has been shown to be effective. More recently, 90 mg fluoxetine weekly (Prozac Weekly) had shown to be an effective and safe treatment (Manasia et al. 2003). Other SSRIs such as sertraline, and paroxetine have been used as well. Adding Sildenafil to Paroxetine had shown to be effective in patients where the Paroxetine alone failed to reverse PE (Chen et al. 2003 and Solania 2002). Generally, SSRIs have fewer adverse effects than tricyclic antidepressants but they carry the risk of caus-ing decreased sexual desire.

2) Tricyclic antidepressants (TCAs): The TCA most stud-ied for PE is clomipramine (Anafranil). Numerous studies showed that clomipramine is more effective for PE than SSRIs in prolonging intra-vaginal latency up to 11 minutes versus up to 6 minutes for fluoxetine, paroxetine or sertra-line. Clomipramine's antidepressant properties are related to its inhibition of the uptake of both norepinephrine and serotonin. Inhibition of serotonin is linked to inhibition of ejaculation. Adult Dose: 50 mg 2–12 h PO before sexual relations; alternatively, 50 mg/d PO once a day.

3) Topical anesthetic agents (TAAs): TAAs decrease penile excitability leading to delayed ejaculations with no adverse

systemic effects. Lidocaine 2.5% and prilocaine 2.5% (EMLA Cream) has been used with significant safety and effectiveness. EMLA Cream is applied to entire penile skin 1–2 hours before sexual intercourse (Berkovitch et al. 1995). SS-cream, a topical cream based on the traditional Chinese Royal Herb Remedy that consists of 9 kinds of natural products (not available in the US) was studied in pilot trials and had shown safety and effectiveness (Xin, Choi, Lee, & Choi, 1997). TAAs side effects of TAAs include erectile problems that could be reduced by applying lesser amounts or restricting the cream to the glans penis. Mouthwash such as Chloraseptic has been shown to be a widely available, safe and effective (Baum and Spieler 2001).

4) Phosphodiesterase 5 inhibitors: Reviews of the literature on the effect of PDE–5 inhibitors on PE revealed that there is benefit from their use due to modulation of the contractile response of the vas deferens, seminal vesicles, prostate and urethra resulting in ejaculatory delays (Abdel-Hamid 2004). Sildenafil, vardenafil, and tadalafil could all be used in the same dosing regimen as prescribed for erectile dysfunction to treat PE either as sole agents or combined with SSRIs.

5) Herbal treatments: Naturopaths use an extract of the herb Passiflora coerulea, known as chrysin (e.g., in Deferol), to produce anti-anxiety effects through the same receptors as the ones diazepam (Valium®) uses. Of course, it's a natural product (bioflavinoid) that does not cause sedation or muscle relaxation. This herb is widely used among body builders, in very high doses, to maximize the effects of testosterone precursors or anabolic steroids (Steidle 2003). More details are provided in Chapter 9 on Alternative Medicine in Sexual Performance Enhancement.

d. No recommended surgical treatment exists for PE

**3. Psychosocial treatments:**

a. General: Including the partner is crucial in the assessment and treatment in order to achieve the best outcome.

b. Behavioral therapy:

   1) Start and stop method: The partner should slowly begin stimulation of the male and should stop as soon as the emergence of a feeling of excessive excitement that may inevitably lead to ejaculation. Stopping sexual stimulation for 30 seconds then resuming, seemed to delay ejaculation. The process should be repeated and practiced at least 10 or more times.

   2) Squeeze method: same as start and stop method, but includes gentle squeezing the base of penis before the 30-second stop period. The squeeze is uncomfortable but not painful. Gradually, most males find it helpful to decrease the impending need to ejaculate.

   3) Biofeedback: electrical feedback helps the individual control the muscles involved in ejaculation.

c. Couple therapy and sex therapy: to address interpersonal and communication problems. The first step for treatment of PE is to relieve any underlying performance pressure on the male. The couple should then be instructed on the start-stop or squeeze techniques introduced by Masters and Johnson. In advanced sensate focus exercises, the couple could practice genito-genital friction with the use of the above techniques, and coitus may be attempted, with the partner on top position so that sexual stimulation could be stopped when ejaculation is impending. Many couples find this to be very successful and serve as an extended foreplay.

d. Individual psychotherapy: aimed at identifying and treating fears and guilt.

### 4. Communication and education

Often the most effective treatment is education. Simply discussing premature ejaculation and its physiology helps men and their partners understand and accurately estimate the issues, and reassures them of the availability of treatment interventions and favorable prognosis.

## F. Prognosis

Masters and Johnson (1970) claimed that the great majority of men with PE (95%) can be treated successfully with the squeeze technique alone within 3 months of the start of therapy although the outcome reported by many practitioners has not been that high. The literature shows that a combination of methods, including medications, with a committed couple generally yield success rates as high as 85%. Relapse rates however are as high as 20–50%, depending on the study. Seftel and Althof (2000) proposed theoretically that medications might be helpful in the short term to regain their sexual confidence, while psychosocial interventions spaced over years would enable couples and individuals to maintain their sexual gains in the long term.

## III. Female Orgasmic Disorder (FOD)

### A. Definition and Phenomenology

As defined below, FOD is the persistent or recurrent delay in, or absence of, orgasm in a female following a normal sexual excitement phase, resulting in marked distress or interpersonal difficulty while it is not better accounted for by another Axis I disorder (apart from other sexual disorders). FOD includes two categories, lifelong anorgasmia (never achieved orgasm) and acquired anorgasmia (has achieved orgasm in past but is no longer able). Women exhibit wide variability in the type or intensity of stimulation that triggers orgasm. The diagnosis of Female Orgasmic Disorder should be based on the clinician's judgment that the woman's orgasmic capacity is less than would be reasonable for her age, menopausal status, sexual experience, and the adequacy of sexual stimulation she receives (APA 2000), in addition to the amount of personal distress the sexual dysfunction has caused.

Women display great variations in orgasmic capacity. The spectrum includes, women who have never had an orgasm, women who become orgasmic only with clitoral self-stimulation when they are alone, women who have orgasms by clitoral stimulation with their partners, women who achieve orgasm during coitus but only after intense clitoral stimulation, women who climax after penetration, and women who can achieve an orgasm solely during non-genital stimulation (i.e., breast, visual, or fantasy stimulation). Additionally, women may also experience multiple orgasms from the various forms of stimulation mentioned above. The percentage of women who achieve orgasm

---

**TABLE 2**

**DSM-IV Diagnostic Criteria for 302.73 Female Orgasmic Disorder**

A. Persistent or recurrent delay in, or absence of, orgasm following a normal sexual excitement phase. Women exhibit wide variability in the type or intensity of stimulation that triggers orgasm. The diagnosis of Female Orgasmic Disorder should be based on the clinician's judgment that the woman's orgasmic capacity is less than would be reasonable for her age, sexual experience, and the adequacy of sexual stimulation she receives.

B. The disturbance causes marked distress or interpersonal difficulty.

C. The orgasmic dysfunction is not better accounted for by another Axis I disorder (except another Sexual Dysfunction) and is not due exclusively to the direct physiological effects of a substance (e.g., a drug of abuse, a medication) or a general medical condition.

Specify type:     Lifelong Type

                  Acquired Type

Specify type:     Generalized Type

                  Situational Type

Specify:          Due to Psychological Factors

                  Due to Combined Factors

Reprinted with permission from the Diagnostic and Statistical Manual of Mental Disorders, Fourth Edition, Text Revision. Copyright 2000 American Psychiatric Association

---

is dependent on the form of stimulation. Only 30% of women regularly achieve orgasm from sexual intercourse, 30% are unable to reach orgasm through sexual intercourse, and 40% have difficulty achieving orgasm from sexual intercourse alone. Therefore, it is essential when evaluating a patient for FOD, the form of stimulation is considered and other sexual techniques or forms of stimulation are explored with the patient (and partner).

Delayed or absence of orgasm could lead to significant personal distress and add a strain to relationships. Types include Life long or acquired, and situational or generalized.

B. **Epidemiology**

In the United States, the National Health and Social Life Survey of 1749 women between the ages of 18 and 59 years revealed that difficulty reaching orgasm is the second most common sexual complaint in women. It has been estimated that approximately 24% of women experience orgasmic difficulties at some point in their lives. The percentage of women experiencing difficulty reaching orgasm declined with age: from 26–28% of 18– to 29–year olds and 30–39-year olds, to 22% and 23% in 40–49 and 50–59 year olds respectively (Laumann et al. 1999). Married women at the time of the survey seemed to have lower rates (22%) compared to never married (30%) and divorced, separated or widowed (32%). The rate of orgasmic difficulties decreased with more education, with college graduates having the lowest rate (18%) and women with less than a high school education having the highest rate (34%).

## C. Etiology

It is very important to rule out the presence of a co-existing sexual disorder at the outset. More significantly, lack of adequate sexual stimulation is a common reason for delayed or absent orgasms. It is crucial for the clinician to evaluate the adequacy of sexual arousal (excitement) before making this diagnosis. Additionally, a comprehensive psychosexual assessment should also be completed to ensure a thorough evaluation of all possible contributing factors.

### 1. Biological factors:

a. General medical conditions such as diabetes and diabetic neuropathy, heart disease, liver disease, kidney disease, multiple sclerosis, and atherosclerosis.

b. Pelvic conditions: Compromised blood flow such as damage to pelvic arteries during surgery, nerve damage due to pelvic surgery or pelvic injury, pelvic floor prolapse, and spinal cord injuries.

c. Alcohol and drugs such as marijuana.

d. Medications are one of the most important etiological factors. SSRIs and benzodiazepines are known to delay or inhibit orgasm.

e. Hormonal changes, often as a result of menopause have been shown to result in diminished sexual responsiveness, decreased genital sensation, and difficulty achieving orgasm (Berman, Berman & Goldstein 1999).

f. Genetic factors are being considered in female orgasmic disorder. A recent study estimated the heritability for difficulty reaching orgasm during intercourse to be 34%, and 45% for orgasm during masturbation (Dunn et al. 2005).

2. **Psychosocial factors:** It is likely that women may commonly experience sexual dysfunction due to psychosocial issues. The presence of poor body and genital image, feelings of low self-esteem, and relationship difficulties all contribute to delayed orgasm and inorgasmia. Positive body image has consistently been demonstrated within the literature to be positively related to more sexual activity, orgasms, and a greater comfort with sexual experiences in general (Ackard, Kearney-Cooke, & Peterson 2000). Genital self-image, defined as the way a woman feels about the size, shape, odor, and function of her genitals (Berman, Berman, Miles, Pollets & Powell 2003) has also been shown to be highly correlated with greater sexual desire, better arousal, lubrication and orgasms, and more satisfaction in her sexual relationships. Research supports the theory that relationship factors may affect sexual experience and function (Berman, Berman, & Goldstein, 1999) and should be considered, especially in women with acquired and situational FOD. For women in particular, emotional functioning and relationship intimacy may be a significant contributor to her physical feelings of sexual satisfaction (Hurlbert, Apt, & Rabehl 1993). Mood disorders, anxiety and other psychological problems may also be interfering with a woman's ability to achieve orgasm (Derogatis, Meyer, & King 1981). Additionally, FOD is strongly and positively correlated with feelings of unhappiness, as well as physical and emotional dissatisfaction (Laumann, Paik, & Rosen 1999). Sexual victimization and an unresolved history of emotional or sexual abuse or trauma are also suggested to increase anorgasmia. Feelings of shame and embarrassment about sexuality as a result of religious beliefs, familial inhibitions, or relationship conflicts may also interfere with orgasm capacity.

Poor sexual technique with ineffective sexual stimulation and an inability to communicate sexual needs and desires have been shown to be related to anorgasmia (Hurlbert 1991). Additionally, the lack of correct anatomic physiological knowledge of the female genitals can increase the potential for sexual dysfunction, particularly in the lack of understanding of female sexual needs and orgasmic triggers (Hoch, Safir, Peres, & Shepher 1981).

## D. Pathophysiology

Central and peripheral mechanisms are involved in delayed or absent orgasm. Central mechanisms include serotonergic and noradrenergic pathways, and supraspinal and spinal circuits. The significance of oxytocin release during orgasm needs further studying in humans. Peripheral mechanisms are heavily in involved in orgasm and require functioning vascular and neuronal infrastructure. Adequacy of sexual stimulation has been generally emphasized. Grafenberg (1950) stated, "An erotic zone always could be demonstrated on the anterior wall of the vagina along the course of the urethra." Named by Ladas, Whipple and Perry (1983) after Dr. Grafenberg as the G-spot, the debate was heated after publication of a review that questioned its anatomical and histological evidence (Hines 2001; Whipple and Perry 2001).

## E. Treatment Approaches:

### 1. Biological interventions:

a. General:

1) Treatment of the underlying medical conditions, whether general or pelvic is key to the success of treatment. Hormonal replacement in cases of hormonal deficiencies is an important step in treatment of FOD.

2) Addressing substances or medications that could lead to delayed or absent orgasm is equally important. Shen et al. (1999) reported that Sildenafil is beneficial in reversing female sexual dysfunction induced by SSRIs. This finding has been replicated in other studies. The reader is referred to Chapter 2 on the Biopsychosocial Evaluation and Treatment of Sexual Disorders for more details on strategies to treat SSRI-induced sexual dysfunction.

b. Physical:

1) Eros therapy: EROS-CTD is a small, handheld medical vacuum device that works by increasing blood flow to the

clitoris and external genitalia. Studies showed improvement in pre- and post-menopausal women with female orgasmic disorder (Billups et al. 2001).

2) Sacral neuromodulation using InterStim® neurostimulator implantation is a reversible treatment that uses mild electrical pulses to stimulate S2, S3 and S4 sacral nerves that contribute to the bladder, sphincter and pelvic floor muscles. Women who received the implant due to urinary bladder control problems reported sexual functioning improvement.

3) Kegel's exercises strengthen voluntary control of the pubo-coccygeus muscle. The muscle is contracted 10–15 times three times per day. Perivaginal muscle tone is expected to improve in 3 months leading to improvement of control and quality of orgasm.

4) Physical exercise

c. Medications: There has been little evidence supporting the use of medications to facilitate orgasm, and treat delayed or absent orgasm. However, recent promising results have been shown with timed doses of long acting dopaminergic agents such as cabergoline prior to intercourse in both normoprolactinemic and hyperprolactinemic individuals (Melmed, IsHak & Berman 2005).

2. **Psychosocial interventions:**

a. General: Including the partner in the assessment and treatment is crucial in order to achieve the best outcome.

b. Psychodynamic psychotherapy: individual therapy sessions to discover and resolve underlying conflicts about orgasm and sexuality. Additionally, for women with secondary anorgasmia, issues relating to trust, safety, and intimacy must be explored in individual therapy. Addressing both negative body & genital self-image within a therapeutic setting is recommended as research has shown that both can significantly impact the ability for a woman to achieve orgasm. Therefore, exploring the patient's self-esteem and sexual image, what messages she has received about her body and genitals and how these are integrated into her self-image, as well as how her negative experience of her body and genitals in impacting her sexual health and functioning.

c. Cognitive behavioral therapy and behavioral therapy:

Cognitive behavioral therapy and behavioral therapy for depression, and anxiety disorders, as well as sexual dysfunction (FOD). CBT has been shown to be effective in treating anorgasmia, and may include decreasing anxiety, changing maladaptive thoughts and attitudes about sexuality, and increasing orgasmic ability and satisfaction (Meston, Hull, Levin, & Sipski, 2004). Focus on behavioral exercises includes directed masturbation, sensate focus, and systematic desensitization. The following three modalities are utilized:

1) Individual CBT

2) Group CBT

3) Biofeedback

d. Directed masturbation is a technique whereby the woman is educated as to how she can induce orgasm. By increasing body-awareness, this knowledge and experience could be applied to sexual intercourse with her partner.

e. Use of internal and external vibrators to help facilitate arousal and orgasm, particularly in women who experience a lack of genital sensation and may need more direct and intense stimulation.

f. Couple therapy and sex therapy: to address interpersonal and communication problems. A variety of issues may be interfering with the relationship including, trust and safety, childrearing, family relationships, or general stress. It is important that these issues are thoroughly explored to better understand their impact on the sexual relationship. Masters and Johnson sensate focus exercises are the main stay behavioral treatment in addition to education and facilitation of communication. Additionally, incorporating sex education and employing specific sexual techniques may be particularly effective when working with a woman with secondary anorgasmia and her partner.

g. For more details the reader is referred to Chapter 2 on the Biopsychosocial Evaluation and Treatment of Sexual Disorders for more details on the technique of Sex Therapy.

h. Focus on women's sexual health issues: More details are provided in Chapter 10 on Women's Sexual Health.

## F. Prognosis

The prognosis depends on whether FOD is lifelong or acquired and whether it is generalized or situational. Research data supports that situational and acquired FOD have better prognosis except in cases where there is permanent pelvic vascular or nerve damage. Further research is needed to better understand how physical, psychological, and relational factors affect orgasm in women.

## IV. Male Orgasmic Disorder (MOD)

### A. Definition and Phenomenology

As defined below, it is the persistent or recurrent delay in, or absence of, orgasm following a normal sexual excitement phase during sexual activity that the clinician, taking into account the person's age, judges to be adequate in focus, intensity, and duration, resulting in marked distress or interpersonal difficulty while it is not better accounted for by another Axis I disorder (apart from other sexual disorders) (APA 2000).

Some men presenting to sexual medicine clinics seek treatment for delayed orgasm. MOD is diagnosed when the delay or absence of orgasm lead to significant personal distress and add strain to relationships. MOD Types include Life long or acquired, and situational or generalized.

### B. Epidemiology

In the United States, the National Health and Social Life Survey of 1410 men between the ages of 18 and 59 years revealed that inability to achieve orgasm is the least common sexual complaint in men. It has been estimated that approximately 8% of men experience orgasmic difficulties at some point in their lives. The percentage of men experiencing inability

---

**TABLE 3**
**DSM-IV Diagnostic Criteria for 302.74 Male Orgasmic Disorder**

A. Persistent or recurrent delay in, or absence of, orgasm following a normal sexual excitement phase during sexual activity that the clinician, taking into account the person's age, judges to be adequate in focus, intensity, and duration.

B. The disturbance causes marked distress or interpersonal difficulty.

C. The orgasmic dysfunction is not better accounted for by another Axis I disorder (except another Sexual Dysfunction) and is not due exclusively to the direct physiological effects of a substance (e.g., a drug of abuse, a medication) or a general medical condition.

Specify type:    Lifelong Type
                 Acquired Type
Specify type:    Generalized Type
                 Situational Type
Specify:         Due to Psychological Factors
                 Due to Combined Factors

Reprinted with permission from the Diagnostic and Statistical Manual of Mental Disorders, Fourth Edition, Text Revision. Copyright 2000 American Psychiatric Association

---

to achieve orgasm did not vary significantly with age, marital status, race or ethnicity. There was a difference in rates between in college graduates (7%) and less than high school education subjects (11%).

## C.  Etiology

Retrograde ejaculation (see Section V) needs to be excluded, as it is a common reason of perceived MOD. Low testosterone levels have been implicated in men with MOD. PTSD and OCD seemed to be more associated with orgasmic disorders in men than women. Thioridazine (Mellaril) has been identified in the literature as a cause of MOD in patients with Schizophrenia (Aizenberg et al. 1996). The rest of the etiological factors of MOD are similar between men and women. Please review the Etiology section on Female Orgasmic Disorder in this chapter.

## D.  Pathophysiology

Central mechanisms have been more implicated in male orgasmic disorder compared to peripheral mechanisms. More studies of the underlying mechanisms of MOD are needed. More details on the physiology of ejaculation are provided in Section II. D.

### E.  Treatment Approaches

#### 1.  Biological interventions:

As described in the previous section, treatment of the underlying medical conditions, hormonal supplementations in cases of hormonal deficiencies, and addressing substances or medications that could lead to delayed or absent orgasm are of prime importance. There was no solid evidence supporting the use of medications to treat MOD until promising results have been shown with timed doses of long acting dopaminergic agents such as cabergoline prior to intercourse in both normoprolactinemic and hyperprolactinemic individuals (Melmed, IsHak & Berman 2005). Cabergoline was administered at 0.5–1 mg. 3–4 hours prior to intercourse. The mechanism of action involving dopamine agonists and prolactin inhibitors is detailed by Kruger et al. (2003). More recently, intra-nasal oxytocin has been used successfully in treatment refractory anorgasmia in a case report (IsHak, Berman and Peters 2007). Oxytocin is administered intra-nasally during intercourse (due to its half-life of 2–3 minutes), at the point when ejaculation is sought. 20–24 IU of Oxytocin delivered through a nasal spray was reported to be effective.

The reader is referred to Chapter 2 on the Biopsychosocial Evaluation and Treatment of Sexual Disorders for more details on strategies to treat SSRI-induced sexual dysfunction.

#### 2.  Psychosocial interventions:

a.  As described in the previous section, important interventions include: engaging the partner in the assessment and treatment, Cognitive Behavioral Therapy and Behavioral Therapy for depressive and anxiety disorders, in addition to Psychodynamic Psychotherapy in order to discover and resolve underlying conflicts about ejaculation and orgasm.

b.  Couple therapy and sex therapy: to address interpersonal and communication problems. The Masters and Johnson sensate focus exercises are the main stay behavioral treatment in addition to education and facilitation of communication. For more details the reader is referred to Chapter 2 on the Biopsychosocial Evaluation and Treatment of Sexual Disorders for more details on the technique of Sex Therapy.

**F. Prognosis**

The prognosis of this condition is largely unknown.

## V. Other Orgasmic Disorders

### Retrograde Ejaculation

Retrograde ejaculation is the condition in which orgasm occurs without the expulsion of fluid and where the fluid had gone backward into the bladder. This condition most commonly occurs in men who have had prostate surgery or in men who have had surgery that resulted in damage to the sympathetic nerves. One of the most common causes is the use of medications. Thioridazine (Mellaril) has been reported in the literature in addition to a small number of case reports on gabapentin (Neurontin). Parasitic infections, venereal diseases, spinal injury, colon cancer surgery, or testicular cancer have been also implicated.

### Orgasmic Cephalgia (sexual headache)

Orgasmic Cephalgia is described as severe headaches reported by women around or after orgasm. Very little is known about this condition that interferes with desire to pursue sexual activity.

## VI. Conclusions and Future Directions

Orgasmic disorders comprise Premature Ejaculation as the most common sexual disorder in men, Female Orgasmic Disorder as the second most common disorder in women, and Male Orgasmic Disorder as the least common sexual disorder in men. Generally, more psychosocial factors are implicated in Premature Ejaculation and Female Orgasmic Disorder compared to Male Orgasmic Disorder where biological and medical factors play an essential role. A variety of behavioral, cognitive, physical, and biological interventions are effective in the treatment. More studies need to be planned to clarify the relationship between sexual stimulation and orgasm especially on the G-spot, and other identified areas linked to increased arousal and orgasm. More studies are needed to clarify central mechanisms controlling orgasmic abilities in both men and women. More trials combining medication and psychotherapy are needed to examine their long-term effectiveness in orgasmic disorder.

# *References*

Abdel-Hamid IA: Phosphodiesterase 5 inhibitors in rapid ejaculation: potential use and possible mechanisms of action. Drugs 64(1):13–26, 2004

Aizenberg D, Shiloh R, Zemishlany Z, Weizman A: Low-dose imipramine for thioridazine-induced male orgasmic disorder. Journal of Sex & Marital Therapy 22(3):225–9, 1996

Ackard DM, Kearney-Cooke A, Peterson CB: Effect of body image and self-image on women's sexual behaviors. International Journal of Eating Disorders 28 (4):422–429, 2000

American Psychiatric Association (APA): Diagnostic and Statistical Manual of Mental Disorders. 4th ed. Text Revision. Washington, DC: American Psychiatric Publishing Inc, 2000

Berman, J.R., Berman, L. & Goldstein, I.: Female sexual dysfunction: incidence, pathophysiology, evaluation, and treatment options. Urology 54:385–391, 1999

Berman L, Berman J, Miles M, Pollets D, & Powell JA: Genital self-image as a component of sexual health: Relationship between genital self-image, female sexual function, and quality of life measures. Journal of Sex & Marital Therapy, 29 (supplement), 11–21, 2003

Billups KL, Berman L, Berman J, et al: A new non-pharmacological vacuum therapy for female sexual dysfunction. J Sex Marital Ther 27(5):435–41, 2001

Chen J, Mabjeesh NJ, Matzkin H, Greenstein A: Efficacy of sildenafil as adjuvant therapy to selective serotonin reuptake inhibitor in alleviating premature ejaculation. Urology 61:197–200, 2003

Chris Steidle, MD, ejaculatory disorders, http://www.seekwellness.com/, 2003

Derogatis LR, Meyer JK and King KM: Psychopathology in individuals with sexual dysfunction. Am J Psychiatry 138:757–763, 1981

Dunn KM, Cherkas LF, Spector TD: Genetic influences on variation in female orgasmic function: a twin study. Biology Letters 1(3):260–263, 2005

Figueira I, Possidente E, Marques C, Hayes K: Sexual dysfunction: a neglected complication of panic disorder and social phobia. Archives of Sexual Behavior 30:369–77, 2001

Grafenberg E: The Role of Urethra in Female Orgasm. The International Journal of Sexology Vol. III, No. 3, p. 145–148, 1950

Grenier G, Byers ES: Operationalizing premature or rapid ejaculation. Journal of Sex Research 38:369–378, 2001

Hines TM: The G-spot: a modern gynecologic myth. American Journal of Obstetrics & Gynecology 185(2):359–62, 2001

Hoch Z, Safir MP, Peres Y, Shepher J: An evaluation of sexual performance—comparison between sexually dysfunctional and functional couples. J Sex Marital Ther. 7(3):195–206, 1981

Hurlbert DF: The role of assertiveness in female sexuality: a comparative study between sexually assertive and sexually nonassertive women. J Sex Marital Ther. 17(3):183–90, 1991

Hurlbert DF, Apt C, Rabehl SM: Key variables to understanding female sexual satisfaction: an examination of women in nondistressed marriages. J Sex Marital Ther. 19(2):154–65, 1993

Kruger TH, Haake P, Haverkamp J, Kramer M, Exton MS, Saller B, Leygraf N, Hartmann U, and Schedlowski M: Effects of acute prolactin manipulation on sexual drive and function in males Journal of Endocrinology 179(3)357–365, 2003

IsHak WW, Berman D, Peters A: Male Anorgasmia Treated with Oxytocin. The Journal of Sexual Medicine (in press).

Ladas AK, Whipple B, Perry DJ: The G-spot and Other Recent Discoveries About Human Sexuality, Bantam Doubleday Dell Publishing Group, New York, NY, 1983

Laumann EO, Paik A, Rosen RC: Sexual dysfunction in the United States: prevalence and predictors. JAMA. 281:537–44, 1999

Manasia P, Pomerol J, Ribe N, et al.: Comparison of the efficacy and safety of 90 mg versus 20 mg fluoxetine in the treatment of premature ejaculation. Journal of Urology 170:164–5, 2003

Masters WH, Johnson VE: Human Sexual Inadequacy. Boston: Littlebrown. 1970.

Melmed S, IsHak WW, Berman D: Use Of Cabergoline For The Treatment of Anorgasmia or Delayed Orgasm, in IsHak WW: Orgasmic Disorders, Sexual Medicine Course. Presented at the American Psychiatric Association annual meeting in Atlanta, GA, May 2005.

Meston CM, Hull E, Levin RJ, Sipski M: Disorders of Orgasm in Women. The Journal of Sexual Medicine 1(1):66, 2004

Michael RT: Sex in America. A definitive survey. Warner Books Inc., 1994

Noble MJ and Lakin M, http://www.emedicine.com/med/topic643.htm, 2002

Salonia A, Maga T, Colombo R, et al.: A prospective study comparing paroxetine alone versus paroxetine plus sildenafil in patients with premature ejaculation. Journal of Urology 168:2486–9, 2002

Screponi E, Carosa E, DiStasi SM, et al.: Prevalence of chronic prostatitis in men with premature ejaculation. Urology 58:198–202, 2001

Seftel AD, Althof SE: Rapid Ejaculation. Current Urology Reports 1:302–306, 2000

Shen WW, Urosevich Z, Clayton DO: Sildenafil in the treatment of female sexual dysfunction induced by selective serotonin reuptake inhibitors. Journal of Reproductive Medicine 44(6):535–42, 1999

Waldinger MD: The neurobiological approach to premature ejaculation. Journal of Urology 168:2359–67, 2002

Waldinger MD: Lifelong premature ejaculation: from authority-based to evidence-based medicine. BJU International. 93:201–7, 2004

Whipple B, Perry JD: The G-spot: a modern gynecologic myth. Comment. American Journal of Obstetrics & Gynecology 187(2):519; author reply 520, 2002

# 8

# Sexual Pain Disorders

MANAR ELBOHY, M.D.

HESHAM SHAFIK, M.D.

WAGUIH WILLIAM ISHAK, M.D.

## I. Introduction

Coital pain is the leading symptom of two major sexual disorders: Dyspareunia and Vaginismus. *The Diagnostic and Statistical Manual of Mental Disorders*, DSM-IV-TR (American Psychiatric Association 2000) lists them as two separate disorders in the subcategory of Sexual Pain Disorders.

### Dyspareunia

Recurrent or persistent genital pain associated with sexual intercourse in either a male or a female, resulting in marked distress or interpersonal difficulty while it is not caused by Vaginismus or lack of lubrication and is not better accounted for by another Axis I disorder (apart from other sexual disorders).

## Vaginismus

Recurrent or persistent involuntary spasm of the musculature of the outer third of the vagina that interferes with sexual intercourse in females, resulting in marked distress or interpersonal difficulty while it is not better accounted for by another Axis I disorder (apart from other sexual disorders).

## Other Sexual Pain Disorders

Chronic Vulvar Pain (not listed in the DSM-IV-TR)

# II. Dyspareunia

## A. Definition and Phenomenology

According to DSM-IV-TR, the diagnosis of Dyspareunia is made when the patient complains of recurrent or persistent genital pain associated with sexual intercourse in either a male or a female, resulting in marked distress or interpersonal difficulty while it is not caused by Vaginismus or lack of lubrication and is not better accounted for by another Axis I disorder (apart from other sexual disorders).

## B. Epidemiology

Dyspareunia is a common complaint in general gynecological practice. Johnson et al. (2004) studied the incidence and prevalence of painful sex. Their data based on the epidemiological catchment's area project, a multistage probability study of the incidence and prevalence of psychiatric disorders in the general population conducted in 1981–83. Only the sample of 3,004 adult community residents in the St. Louis area was queried on DSM-III sexual dysfunctions. They found a prevalence rate of 13% for painful sex.

A previous study was done by Glatt et al. (1990), they sent a questionnaire regarding sexual experience and dyspareunia to 428 women, of whom 313 responders. One hundred twenty-two (39.0%) had never had dyspareunia and 86 (27.5%) had had dyspareunia at some point

**TABLE 1**
**Diagnostic Criteria for 302.76 Dyspareunia**

A. Recurrent or persistent genital pain associated with sexual intercourse in either a male or a female.

B. The disturbance causes marked distress or interpersonal difficulty.

C. The disturbance is not caused exclusively by Vaginismus or lack of lubrication, is not better accounted for by another Axis I disorder (except another Sexual Dysfunction), and is not due exclusively to the direct physiological effects of a substance (e.g., a drug of abuse, a medication) or a general medical condition.

Specify type:    Lifelong Type
                     Acquired Type

Specify type:    Generalized Type
                     Situational Type

Specify:    Due to Psychological Factors
               Due to Combined Factors

Reprinted with permission from the Diagnostic and Statistical Manual of Mental Disorders, Fourth Edition, Text Revision. Copyright 2000 American Psychiatric Association

in their lives that resolved. One hundred five women (33.5%) still had dyspareunia at the time of the survey.

Reviewing different studies, incidence figures vary widely; this wide variation might be due to different methodology, sample selection and the analysis of data. The incidence varied from 3% (Hawton 1982), 11% (Rosen et al. 1993), 30.6% (Gurel and Gurel 1999), to 46% (Jamieson and Steege 1996). In a recent study a total of 3,017 women aged 20–60 participating in a screening program for cervical cancer answered a questionnaire about possible painful coitus. The prevalence was 9.3% for the whole group (Danielsson et al. 2003)

## C. Etiology

Many factors may have impact on the development and maintenance of dyspareunia. Both biological and psychosocial etiology has to be discussed. The etiology of dyspareunia should be viewed on a continuum from primarily physical to primarily psychological with many women falling in the middle area (Sandberg and Quevillon 1987). An understanding of the present organic etiology must be integrated with an appreciation of the ongoing psychological factors and negative expectations and attitudes that perpetuate the pain cycle (Heim 2001).

1. **Biological factors:**

    Any complaint of pain that possibly have a physical cause must be properly investigated. There is a presumed high incidence of physical disease associated with dyspareunia when compared with other female sexual dysfunctions. Physical factors that might be claimed include:

    a. Inflammatory: inflammation of the vulva and interstitial cystitis, infections of the vagina, cervix, fallopian tubes or lower urinary tract. Trichomonas, and mycotic organisms are considered important in this regard (Bancroft 1989).

    b. Abscesses of Bartholin's glands or ducts, and Vulvar vestibulitis that give rise to intensive pain during sexual intercourse (Bohm-Starke and Rylander 2000).

    c. Allergic: allergic reactions to the contents of contraceptive foams and jellies and condoms. The vulva may be inflamed, tender or irritated from using soaps or over-the-counter vaginal sprays or douches.

    d. Hormonal: Estrogen deficiency is a particularly common cause of sexual pain complaints among postmenopausal women (Bachmann et al. 1984). Lactation also causes a hypo-estrogenic state as a result of increased prolactin, which can result in atrophic vaginitis with dryness and thinning of the mucosa. So many lactating women experience dyspareunia as the result of these vaginal changes (Reamy et al.1987).

    e. Dryness: Dryness and lack of moisture are from common causes of pain. Sometimes due to medication that decreases vaginal lubrication (such as antihistamines), as a part of or with certain medical conditions, or because of lack of arousal, or inadequate stimulation may result in inadequate vaginal lubrication and cause coital pain. Dryness can occur at certain times of life such as during or just after pregnancy.

    f. Surgical: tight introitus secondary to plastic repair of the vagina, or perineorrhaphy following episiotomy (Bancroft 1989).

g. Anatomical conditions: Hymenal remnants can contribute to coital discomfort (Sarrell and Sarrell 1989) abnormalities of the female genital tract such as congenital septum, or a rigid hymen.

h. Radiation: Women undergoing radiation therapy for pelvic malignancy often experience severe dyspareunia because of the atrophy of the vaginal walls and their susceptibility to trauma (Heim 2001).

i. Drug use: Dyspareunia is associated with illicit drug use and marijuana use (Johnson et al. 2004).

j. Less common etiologies are endometriosis, pelvic congestion, adhesions and adnexal pathology (Heim 2001).

2. **Psychosocial factors**

Psychosocial factors are infrequently involved as a cause of dyspareunia. Most commonly associated factors are:

a. Stressors: Such as deaths or serious illnesses of self, family, close friends; moves; change in job; addition to family; divorce, break up, marriage, new relationship; pregnancy, miscarriage, abortion; financial changes, legal changes may take a toll on sexual functioning (Heiman 1994). Low income is a risk factor for dyspareunia (Jamieson et al. 1996).

b. Religious values: Because of religious values some woman feel that they do not deserve to experience pleasure (Heiman 1994). Others feel with sin and immorality and those feelings of guilt and fear accompanied early sexual exploration and experimentation (Walker et al. 1988).

c. Previous sexual trauma: Heiman (1994) mentioned that, women with sexually or physical abusive histories suffer sexual dysfunctions especially pain, more often than other women. Patients with long-term sexual abuse by a family member may be particularly difficult to recover. Edward et al. (1992) hypothesized that both social and emotional withdrawal in victims of post-traumatic disorder act as coping mechanisms that enable the patient to avoid stimuli that evoke aversive visual and autonomic memories of trauma. Accordingly patients with dyspareunia may experience the pain as a partial "memory" of the abuse without being consciously aware of the full extent of the memory (i.e. physical, autonomic and emotional traumatic memory of the abuse). This might be an adaptive response that allows the patient to avoid stimulating more complete memories of painful childhood sexual victimization.

d. Unresolved anxieties: Unresolved anxieties regarding parental prohibition of sex, inadequacy as a sexual partner, ambivalence or about an abortion, these are all areas of feelings that can generate a complaint of pain (Montford 1992)

e. Role of woman: Dyspareunia can be related to conscious or unconscious rejection of the role of woman or mother (Duguay 1976).

f. Body image: Poor self-esteem and poor perception of one's body image may also be implicated.

g. Unresolved conflicts which undermine the mutual acceptance that is important to healthy sexual functioning (Metz and Epstein 2002). Satisfaction in relationship and degree of happiness is also important area (Heiman 1994).

## D. Pathophysiology and Differential Diagnosis

Dyspareunia has to be differentiated from other physical or psychological causes of coital pain. The differential diagnoses include inadequate lubrication, atrophy and vulvar vestibulitis that has been increasingly identified as a source of excruciating superficial pain for some women (Marinoff and Turner 1991). Psychosexual factors, such as vaginismus, loss of libido, arousal disorders and sexual pain-related disorders often overlap (Graziottin 2001).

So the clinician's main assessment tool is a careful examination of the condition. Beside that the use of technology will elicit further demonstrable causes. Physical examination may reproduce the pain of different type and site. Heim (2001) demonstrated that localized pain with vulvar vestibulitis induced when the vagina is touched with a cotton swab, or involuntary spasm of vaginismus may be noted with insertion of an examining finger or speculum. While palpation of the lateral vaginal walls, uterus, adnexa and urethral structures helps identify the cause.

Regarding the differentiation between dyspareunia and vaginismus many authors pointed to the difficulty to find useful criteria to distinguish between both entities. A retrospective study was undertaken by van Lankveld et al. (1995) to investigate predictors of vaginismus, dyspareunia and mixed sexual pain disorder in respect of symptom profile and treatment history variables of female patients and their partners. The study sample consisted of 147 female patients attending a university hospital outpatient clinic for Psychosomatic Gynecology and Sexology. All patients met the DSM-III-R criteria of the diagnoses of vaginismus (n = 50), dyspareunia (n = 46), or of both diagnoses (n = 51). No uni-variate differences were found between members of the three groups or between their partners.

Based on both the interview and the physical examination, De Kruiff al. (2000) found no significant differences between patients with vaginismus and dyspareunia, in the ability to insert a finger into the vagina or to have a gynecological examination, also the reported level of pain during coitus, in palpated vaginal muscular tension and reported anxiety or tension during the examination.

Vaginal spasm and pain measures did not differentiate between women in the vaginismus and dyspareunia. However, women in the vaginismus group demonstrated significantly higher vaginal/pelvic muscle tone and lower muscle strength. Also displayed a significantly higher frequency of defensive/avoidant distress behaviors during pelvic examinations and recalled past attempts at intercourse with more affective distress (Reissing al. 2004).

### E. Treatment Approaches

#### 1. Diagnostic work-up:

Once a patient reports dyspareunia, a thorough history taking should help to define the problem and should directed to:

a. Identify the history of the pain, its site, sort, severity, onset, duration, chronology and any other associated factors.

b. Look for any physical abnormalities and discuss their effects on the sexual relationship.

c. Review of earlier attempts to alleviate the dyspareunia.

d. Rule out the other causes of coital pain.

e. Gynecological, urological, and neurological consultations and full work-up.

f. Psychiatric work-up should include ruling out disorders that might be related to dyspareunia such as depressive, anxiety and somatoform disorders.

g. Keep in mind common theories of etiology of sexual dysfunction (Steege 1984)

h. Assessment instruments include the Visual Analogue for pain (scale from 0 to 10, the latter being the most severe pain).

2. **Biological and physical treatments:**

a. Treatment of underlying medical conditions:

Treatment of dyspareunia should be directed first, at underlying causes (Walton and Thorton 2003). Therapy for an underlying cause may be as simple as prescribing antibiotics for vaginal infection, and adjunctive therapy for menopausal women, as use of lubricants and estrogen containing creams or may involve hormonal or surgical therapy for endometriosis or congenital anomalies. For some patients with pelvic pain, the exclusion of a physical cause may come as an emotional relief with subsequent relief from pain (Montford 1992), while others, reassurance without exploring the fantasy is not enough. Sometimes the examination or investigations itself particularly when painful may increase or be the cause of more persistent pain.

b. Physical interventions:

Leiblum (1995) mentioned that, training in progressive muscle relaxation, as well as instruction in Kegel exercises, masturbation can be suggested as well as self-stimulation as this enables the woman to become desensitized to touching her genitalia. Huffman (1992) suggested the de-conditioning by vaginal dilators. Various audiovisual materials can be used in the treatment. The results of several studies suggest that sexually explicit materials may have some desensitizing effects when used in a graduated fashion under the control of individuals who can terminate the stimuli in response to their anxiety level

(Neidigh and Kinder 1987). However, it appears that the use of such materials may actually lead to increases in anxiety if used in an indiscriminate way.

c. Electrical stimulation (ES): Nappi et al. (2003) investigated the use of (ES) on the vestibular area and vaginal introitus in women with sexual pain disorders. They evaluated the muscular activity of the perineal floor and sexual function, and evaluated pain. Major findings were as follows: the contractile ability of pelvic floor muscles as well as the resting ability significantly improved following ES; the pain significantly declined. They found that following (ES) four out of nine women with vaginismus went back to coital activity.

d. Ultrasound: Based on trial, women treated with ultrasound for persistent perineal pain and/or dyspareunia were less likely to report pain with sexual intercourse compared with the placebo group There is not enough evidence to evaluate the use of ultrasound in treating perineal pain and/or dyspareunia following childbirth (Hay-Smith 2000).

e. Pelvic-relaxation exercises (combined with education and counseling) may be needed to restore the woman's confidence and decrease anxiety (Sarazin and Seymour 1991).

f. Medications:

Analgesics might be helpful for temporary treatment of dyspareunia. Topical nitroglycerin was shown to be safe and effective in introital dyspareunia and vulvar pain in women with vulvodynia. 0.2% nitroglycerin cream was applied to the skin at the genital/vulvar area where the pain was located 5–10 minutes prior to sexual relations (Walsh et al. 2002).

3. **Psychosocial treatments:**

a. General:

Before psychiatric intervention all organic causes of dyspareunia should be ruled out first. Montford (1992) advised the use an unstructured Interview, and to allow the patient to choose the topic for discussion. Then, by observing the patient's attitude to examination, clues to the patient's real distress may be picked up. Walton and Thorton( 2003) confirmed that, an open discussion about relational, situational, and psychological issues should be done to address the exact sexual dysfunction (Walton and Thorton 2003)

b. Sex therapy:

Different modalities of treatment can be applied, cognitive sex therapy that is viewed as a process of script modification can facilitate the occurrence of a sexual act (Gagnon et al. 1982). Discussion of the cognitive beliefs and assumptions the patient holds about sex and challenging unrealistic or unexplored cognitive beliefs and assumptions enables female patients to reassess and "update" their sexual values (Leiblum 1995). Script modification places a particular emphasis on the cognitive and interpersonal dimensions of sexual interaction. Clinical assessment of sexual scripts begins with a comparison of performative and cognitive scripts, which are then elaborated in terms of key script attributes such as complexity, rigidity, conventionality and satisfaction (Gagnon et al. 1982).

Simon and Gagnon (1986) explained that the scripting of behavior is examined on three distinct levels: cultural scenarios, interpersonal scripts and intrapsychic scripts. These concepts of the scripting of behavior are then applied to sexual behavior.

On the other side the basic principles of behaviorists' approaches are treatment of the couple and mutual involvement of both partners. Gellman (1983) aiming to eliminate sexual anxieties, changing negative attitudes toward sexuality and improving of verbal and corporal communication within the couple. Author suggested that sexual information and education (regarding the cycle of sexual response, anatomy, biology), and sexual techniques, learning to know one self and others better could help.

c. Couple therapy:

Regarding couples that presenting for sex therapy and has difficulties in resolving conflict and in expressing emotional as well as physical intimacy. Russell (1990) has shown that intimacy is an important variable in determining the health or pathology in the dyadic system. Furthermore, the level of intimacy is influenced by a capacity for self-disclosure and an ability to consider the partner's opinion. Encourages self-disclosure to facilitate mutual understanding, decrease conflict, and increase intimacy.

d. Hypnosis:

Although hypnosis has been suggested as treatment for dyspareunia, but empirical data and case reports showing its effectiveness have been lacking. Kandyba and Binik (2003) have shown the effect of hypnotherapy in a case study, a 26-year-old woman suffering from dyspareunia. Psychotherapy consisted of twelve sessions; of which eight were devoted to hypnosis was done. They found that the patient experienced no more pain following treatment, and remained pain free at a 12-month follow up. They explained that, hypnosis help to decrease of anticipatory anxiety, create a positive association of pleasure with intercourse, and create a sense of control over her pain.

4. **Communication and education:**

Effective treatment of dyspareunia can be a simple matter of reassuring the patient or conferring with her sexual partner (Huffman 1976). While dyspareunia of long standing or more complicated relationship may require different approaches. Hence, Integrated treatment approaches have been developed, as cognitive-behavioral and couples' therapy procedures are increasingly combined with traditional sex therapy techniques (Rosen and Leiblum 1995). Sex education and engagement of the couple in the process is of prime importance in dyspareunia.

F. **Prognosis**

Although treatment for dyspareunia is rarely straightforward and brief, significant progress can be achieved and therapeutic outcome can be quite positive (Leiblum 1995). Steege and Ling (1993) Mentioned that Dyspareunia that occurs after a period of good sexual adjustment may be more amenable to an office-based counseling and educational approach, assuming that the patient and her partner are comfortable and cooperative in approaching the problem. While Dyspareunia of long standing or in a more complicated relationship may require skills possessed by more highly trained professionals.

## III. Vaginismus

### A. Definition and Phenomenology

According to DSM-IV-TR (American Psychiatric Association 2000), the essential feature of Vaginismus is the recurrent or persistent involuntary spasm of the musculature of the outer third of the vagina that interferes with sexual intercourse in females, resulting in marked distress or interpersonal difficulty while it is not better accounted for by another Axis I disorder (apart from other sexual disorders).

The woman who experiences involuntary, spasmodic contraction of the pubococcygeus and related muscles controlling the vaginal introitus may be unable to tolerate penetration or have intercourse, but may be quite capable of becoming sexually aroused, lubricating, and even experiencing multiple orgasms with manual or oral stimulation (Leiblum et al. 1989). This spasm is produced by imagined or real attempts at vaginal penetration (Dennerstein and Burrows 1977).

### B. Epidemiology

Despite vaginismus is one of the common female psychosexual problems, very limited data on the incidence and prevalence of vaginismus

---

**TABLE 2**
**Diagnostic Criteria for 306.51 Vaginismus**

A. Recurrent or persistent involuntary spasm of the musculature of the outer third of the vagina that interferes with sexual intercourse.

B. The disturbance causes marked distress or interpersonal difficulty.

C. The disturbance is not better accounted for by another Axis I disorder (e.g., Somatization Disorder) and is not due exclusively to the direct physiological effects of a general medical condition.

Specify type:    Lifelong Type
                 Acquired Type
Specify type:    Generalized Type
                 Situational Type
Specify:         Due to Psychological Factors
                 Due to Combined Factors

Reprinted with permission from the Diagnostic and Statistical Manual of Mental Disorders, Fourth Edition, Text Revision. Copyright 2000 American Psychiatric Association

are available. Reviewing some of the previous studies, figures regarding the incidence of vaginismus are varying widely. Vaginismus rates have been reported ranging between 12% and 17% of females presenting to sexual therapy clinics (Spector and Carey 1990). While O'Sullivan (1979), describes a group of 23 Irish women with vaginismus. This figure represents 42% of the total female referrals to the author, which is quite high when compared with other reports. So till now there is lacking for sufficient, significant epidemiological studies regarding both the prevalence and the incident of vaginismus.

## C. Etiology

### 1. Biological factors:

Concerning etiological correlates of vaginismus, rarely physical abnormalities may be present; most cases of vaginismus are caused by emotional or psychological factors. Vaginismus appears to be a somatic manifestation of unconscious psychological conflicts. Even the causes of vaginismus seem to vary and are not fully understood.

### 2. Psychosocial factors:

There are several theories as to what those psychological causes are, but most centers around:

a. Past sexual trauma: Some women with vaginismus have a history of sexual abuse, rape or other trauma and have an intense fear of further pain, penetration or violation. Most of the women with vaginismus either witnessed or experienced actual physical violation in their histories (Silverstein 1989). Such experience of physical or sexual abuse can induce phobia of vaginal penetration. Reissing et al. (2003) mentioned that, some women with vaginismus reported a history of childhood sexual interference, and women in both the vaginismus and dyspareunia groups reported lower levels of sexual functioning and a less positive sexual self-schema.

b. Sometimes women with vaginismus perceive the vaginal penetration as violation or invasion. The symptom serves to protect against violation. The tightening of the pelvic muscles may be an unconscious effort by these women to protect them. Other causes are fear of being controlled by a man, of losing control, or of being hurt during coitus.

c. Developmental factors: Some authors suggested that high moral expectations instilled by the mother (Barnes, 1986), negative psychosexual upbringing, religious taboos that invest sex with shame and guilt and religious upbringing (Silverstein, 1989), intrapsychic fears and conflicts may be blamed. Silverstein (1989) examined family patterns of 22 women seeking psychotherapy for vaginismus due to psychosocial reasons. It was found that nearly all of the women had domineering, threatening fathers who were moralistic but also sexually seductive. The parents of these women had high levels of conflict and verbal and/or physical abuse in their marriages. The women with vaginismus were the 'good girls' of their families, obedient, unable to express anger and in constant need of approval. Both the women and their partners fear aggression.

d. Conditioned association of pain/fear with vaginal penetration: Kaplan (1974) suggested a view of vaginismus as a conditioned response to any adverse stimulus associated with intercourse or vaginal entry. Reissing et al. (1999) propose a re-conceptualization of vaginismus as either an aversion/phobia of vaginal penetration or a genital pain disorder.

Leiblum (1995) stated that, behavioral therapists generally view vaginismus as a conditioned fear reaction or a learned phobia. Reinforcing the conditioned fear response is the cognitive belief that penetration can be accomplished only with great difficulty, pain, and discomfort.

e. Psychoanalytic explanations: Leiblum (1995) gave a historical, psychoanalytic explanations of vaginismus, that the disorder was conceived of as a rejection of the female role, or resistance against male sexual prerogative, a defense of the woman against her father's real or fantasized incestual threats, or a warding off of a woman's own castration images (Fenichel 1945).

f. Relational factors: As it is mentioned before relationship deficiencies, such as undermine the mutual acceptance is important to healthy sexual functioning (Metz and Epstein 2002) unre-solved conflict or feeling emotionally abused by her partner might be claimed. Leiblum (1995) Mentioned that a partner's sexual clumsiness, conflicted and antagonistic feelings toward men in general, or one's sexual partner in particular, may be an etiological factor. While Silverstein (1989) found that, these women tend to choose partners who appear to be the opposite of their fathers; they seem kind, gentle and often passive.

g. Secondary type of vaginismus (which occurring after a period of normal sexual function) is common. If women have experienced vaginal pain caused by new onset of infection, surgical or post delivery scarring, Endometriosis, Inadequate vaginal lubrication.

## D. Pathophysiology

van der Velde and Everaerd (1999) tried to differentiate between women with and without vaginistic reactions regarding the ability to voluntarily contract and relax the pelvic floor muscles. Using intravaginal surface electromyographic (EMG) recordings of the pelvic floor muscles and EMG measurements of the surrounding muscle groups, during muscle exercises. They found no difference in baseline and performance of the exercises between groups, indicating a comparable level of relaxation. They concluded that the women with vaginistic reactions do not have less voluntary control. In more recent study, van der Velde et al. (2001) mentioned that the increase in muscle activity is not restricted to the pelvic floor but will also occur in postural muscles, such as in the trapezius region. Exposure to a threatening situation will evoke an increase in muscle activity. They found that this increase of involuntary pelvic floor muscle activity is part of a general defense mechanism that occurs during exposure to threatening situations. This reaction is not restricted to a situation with a sexual content. Shafik and El-Sibai (2002) studied the EMG activity of the levator ani (LA), puborectalis (PR) and bulbocavernosus (BC) muscles, to define the involved muscles and their role in the pathogenesis of vaginismus. In their case control study, they found that the pelvic floor muscles of vaginismus patients exhibited increased EMG activity at rest and on vaginismus induction. They suggested that the concept of a disordered sacral reflex arc is put forward but needs further studies to be verified.

### E. Treatment Approaches

Treatment aims at helping the woman to regain voluntary control of her pelvic floor muscles Biswas and Ratnam (1995). Treatment methods of vaginismus range from surgery, simple muscle strengthening exercises to elaborate psychotherapeutic intervention. More recently, behavioral methods have shown marked success. The most important considerations in therapy seem to be the patient's understanding of the problem and flexibility of approach (Fertel 1977).

1. **Diagnostic work-up**

   a. Clarify details of vaginismus, and the presence of pain if any.

   b. Gynecological, urological, and neurological consultations.

   c. Psychiatric work-up should include ruling out disorders that might be related to vaginismus such as anxiety and somatoform disorders.

2. **Biological and physical treatments**

   a. Relaxation, self and mutual pleasuring exercises, Control of vaginal muscles, Kegel exercises, and self-exploration of sexual anatomy all have shown usefulness as therapeutic tools.

   b. Systemic desensitization: Vaginismus, as a reaction of avoidance of an anxiety-producing situation, is readily amenable to treatment by systematic desensitization. Becker and Kavoussi (1994) mentioned that systematic desensitization has been the most effective treatment method for vaginismus. They described the procedure that involves systematic insertion of dilators of graduated sizes, either in the doctor's office or in the privacy of the patient's home. When digital vaginal dilatation can be painlessly carried out, intercourse is attempted (Dennerstein and Burrows 1977). Biswas and Ratnam (1995) proposed two approaches to vaginal desensitization: The first is gradual desensitization using vaginal self-dilatation, and the second method utilizes rapid desensitization brought about by vaginal mould insertion. Management of these conditions requires a warm, empathetic attitude and demands great patience and understanding on the part of the physician. Fuchs (1980) suggested that desensitization might proceed mainly in two ways: "in vitro" or "in vivo."

In order to strengthen and speed up the desensitization process, use of hypnotic techniques in a dynamic approach. The "in vitro" treatment proceeds with imagery, under hypnosis, of an "anxiety hierarchy" of increasingly erotic and sexually intimate situations, which will be reproduced at home with the partner, until sexual intercourse is achieved. In the "in vivo" method the patient learns self-hypnosis and then inserts in the vagina first a finger, and then Hegar dilators of gradually increasing sizes. The partner, the patient, and the physician will then successively proceed to insertion, forming a team-referred work situation. This continues until the "female superior position," practiced first with the largest dilator, is reproduced at home by intercourse.

c. Medications:

Although there are no specific medication interventions for vaginismus, the use of intravenous diazepam abreaction interviews was reported. Mikhail (1976) interviewed four patients between the ages of 19 and 28. The duration of their main complaint varied from 6 months to 3 years. Three to six abreaction interviews were conducted. All of these patients reported having successful intercourse after these interviews. Individual psychotherapy continued after the interviews on a weekly basis, and marital therapy on a monthly basis, for a period of 2 to 6 months. Three out of four women reported being orgasmic for the first time. Kaplan et al. (1982) studied case histories of three patients with sexual phobias. All had been treatment failures with sex therapy and psychotherapy but responded to a combination of tricyclic medication and sex therapy, which was modified to accommodate the special needs of sexually phobic patients. Botulinium toxin (Botox) have been used successfully in this condition. See Chapter 4 Section VI B for more details.

3. **Psychosocial treatments**

a. Psychodynamic psychotherapy: In some women, vaginismus appears to be a somatic manifestation of unconscious psychological conflicts. These women may benefit from more intensive psychotherapy (Dennerstein and Burrows 1977).

b. Cognitive-behavioral psychotherapy: Leiblum (1995) suggested that, the inappropriate cognitions about the size of the vagina, the size of the penis, and the likelihood of pain must be challenged. Kabakci and Batur (2003) found that all of the participants were treated effectively by cognitive-behavioral therapy (CBT). By the end of the therapy, anxiety levels of the women decreased. There also were improvements on parameters related to marital harmony and overall sexual functioning of the women. Shaw (1994) challenged the efficacy of a cognitive-behavioral treatment model for women with primary vaginismus and proposes a conceptual shift from a focus on behavior to a focus on differentiation. Primary vaginismus is viewed as a somatic boundary, a symbolic description of an opportunity for differentiation. Four relevant themes are considered: 1) mastery versus incompetence; 2) autonomy versus dependence; 3) boundary versus fusion; and 4) the effect on the therapy of the therapist's level of differentiation. Change at this particular time in history involves shifts in clinical focus from sexual frequency to quality, from performance to experience, from compliance to mastery, and from utilization function to sexual potential.

c. Behavioral therapy: Some studies examined the use of biofeedback as an adjunct to psychotherapy in the treatment of vaginismus. Barnes et al. (1984) concluded that biofeedback is an effective aid to learning muscle control, is acceptable to patients, and may increase the success.

d. Sex therapy and couple therapy: Sex therapy aims at refocusing the couple on pleasure as a main theme in sexual activity. Engaging the couple in sensate focus exercises help shift the focus from penetration and the concerns of having vaginismus to more of a relaxed mutually pleasurable mode. Couple therapy help address some of the communication problems that are deemed to interfere with improvement in the sexual relationship. Sex therapy techniques is discussed in more details in Chapter 2 on Biopsychosocial Evaluation and Treatment of Sexual Disorders.

e. Bibliotherapy conveys the therapeutic interventions without the physical presence of a therapist using educational materials, literature, and workbooks. van Lankveld published a meta-analysis of Cognitive-behavioral bibliotherapy concluding that it leads to positive results at the end of a brief treatment period of patients with sexual dysfunction especially vaginismus with minimal therapist support (van Lankveld 1998).

### 4. Communication and education

The most important considerations in therapy seem to be the patient's understanding of the problem and flexibility of approach (Fertel1977). Sexual education of the couple plays an important role in understanding some of the issues surrounding Vaginismus.

## F. Prognosis

Scholl (1988) followed up Twenty-three patients with vaginismus in a Sexual Dysfunction Program over five years. Twenty of these patients continued in therapy and had successful outcomes. This follow-up study has demonstrated that the maintenance of treatment gains over time for most women. Lamont (1978) mentioned that, with the use of the combination of available techniques, good success could be obtained in treating vaginismus with the conjoint approach or office management of the woman alone. Kabakci and Batur (2003) investigated a group of Turkish vaginismus patients who benefited from CBT. They found that all of the participants were treated effectively by CBT. Mikhail (1976) interviewed four patients and reported all of these patients having successful intercourse after using intravenous diazepam abreaction interviews. Schnyder et al. (1998) in their study to assess the effectiveness of desensitization exercises in the treatment of vaginismus. They found that Forty-three (97.2%) of the patients were able to have sexual intercourse. So outcome data, vary dramatically from one study to another, and vary by the use of different ways of treatment.

# IV. Other Sexual Pain Disorders

Chronic Vulvar Pain is a significant sexual pain complaint that is not listed as a disorder in the DSM-IV-TR classification. Causes of chronic vulvar pain such as vulvodynia; cyclic vulvovaginitis, and other medical and psychological causes are discussed in details in Chapter 10 on Women's Sexual Health.

## V. Conclusion and Future Directions

Sexual Pain Disorders namely Dyspareunia and Vaginismus are clinically significant medical/psychological problems. Generally, more biological factors are implicated in dyspareunia, while more psychosocial factors are implicated in vaginismus. Treatment of underlying medical conditions is an essential part in the treatment of Sexual Pain Disorders in addition to psychosocial interventions in the form of individual psychotherapy and/or sex therapy. The importance of education and working with the couple cannot be overemphasized. More studies need to be planned to clarify some basic confusions between the nature of dyspareunia and vaginismus as detailed in Section II. D. More studies are needed to examine the relationship between dyspareunia and somatoform disorders as well as understanding the biological and psychosocial underpinnings of vaginismus e.g., concepts such as a disordered sacral reflex arc in vaginismus.

## *References*

American Psychiatric Association (APA): Diagnostic and Statistical Manual of Mental Disorders, 4th Edition. Text Revision Washington, DC: American Psychiatric Publishing Inc, 2000

Barnes J, Bowman EP, Cullen J: Biofeedback as an adjunct to psychotherapy in the treatment of vaginismus. Biofeedback Self Regul. Sep; 9(3): 281–9, 1984

Binik YM, Reissing E, Pukall C, Flory N, Payne KA, Khalife S: The female sexual pain disorders: genital pain or sexual dysfunction? : Arch Sex Behav. Oct; 31(5): 425–9, 2002

Biswas A, Ratnam SS: Vaginismus and outcome of treatment. Ann Acad Med Singapore Sep; 24(5): 755–8, 1995

Bohm-Starke N, Rylander E: Vulvar vestibulitis is a condition with diffuse etiology. Lakartidningen 97(43): 4832–6, 2000

Clemens JQ, Nadler RB, Schaeffer AJ et al.: Biofeedback, pelvic floor re-education, and bladder training for male chronic pelvic pain syndrome. Urology 56(6): 951–5, 2000

Danielsson I, Sjoberg I, Stenlund H, Wikman M: Prevalence and incidence of prolonged and severe dyspareunia in women: results from a population study. Scand J Public Health 31(2):113–8, 2003

de Kruiff ME, ter Kuile MM, Weijenborg PT, van Lankveld JJ: Vaginismus and dyspareunia: is there a difference in clinical presentation? J Psychosom Obstet Gynaecol. 21(3): 149–55, 2000

Dennerstein L, Burrows GD: The management of vaginismus. Aust Fam Physician 6(12):1545–9, 1977

DeWitt DE: Dyspareunia. Tracing the cause. Postgrad Med. 89(5): 67–8, 70, 73, 1991

Duguay R: Sexual dysfunctions of emotional origin in women. Union Med Can. 105(12): 1849–51, 1976

Fertel NS: Vaginismus: a review. J Sex Marital Ther. 3(2): 113–21, 1977

Fuchs K: Therapy of vaginismus by hypnotic desensitization. Am J Obstet Gynecol. 137(1): 1–7, 1980

Gagnon JH, Rosen RC, Leiblum SR: Cognitive and social aspects of sexual dysfunction: sexual scripts in sex therapy. J Sex Marital Ther.8(1): 44–56, 1982
Graziottin A: Clinical approach to dyspareunia. J Sex Marital Ther. 27(5): 489–501, 2001

Glatt A, Zinner S, McCormack W: The prevalence of dyspareunia. Obstet Gynecol. 75:433–436, 1990

Gurel H, Atar Gurel S: Dyspareunia, back pain and chronic pelvic pain: the importance of this pain complex in gynecological practice and its relation with grandmultiparity and pelvic relaxation. Gynecol Obstet Invest. 48 (2): 119–22, 1999

Gutl P, Greimel ER, Roth R, Winter R: Women's sexual behavior, body image and satisfaction with surgical outcomes after hysterectomy: a comparison of vaginal and abdominal surgery. Psychosom Obstet Gynaecol. 23(1): 51–9, 2002

Hawton K: The behavioral treatment of sexual dysfunction. Br J Psychiatry 140:94–101, 1982

Hay-Smith EJ: Therapeutic ultrasound for postpartum perineal pain and dyspareunia. Cochrane Database Syst Rev.(2): CD0004, 2000

Heim LJ: Etiology and diagnosis of coital pain. J Endocrinol Invest. 26(3 Suppl): 115–21, 2003

Heim LJ: Evaluation and differential diagnosis of dyspareunia. Am Fam
     Physician 63(8): 1535–44, 2001

Heiman JR: Female sexual dysfunction. In Singer C, Weiner WJ, (eds): Sexual
     Dysfunction: A Neuro-Medical Approach. Armonk, NY: Futura
     Publishing Company, Inc, 1994

Heiman JR: Psychologic treatments for female sexual dysfunction: are they
     effective and do we need them? Arch Sex Behav. 31(5): 445–50, 2002

Huffman JW: Dyspareunia of vulvo-vaginal origin. Causes and management.
     Postgrad Med. 73(2): 287–96, 1983

Jamieson DJ, Steege JF: The prevalence of dysmenorrhea, dyspareunia, pelvic
     pain, and irritable bowel syndrome in primary care practices. Obstet
     Gynecol. 87(1): 55–8, 1996

Johnson SD, Phelps DL, Cottler LB: The association of sexual dysfunction and
     substance use among a community epidemiological sample. Arch Sex
     Behav. Feb; 33(1): 55–63, 2004
     Kabakci E, Batur S: Who benefits from cognitive behavioral therapy
     for vaginismus? J Sex Marital Ther. 29(4): 277–88, 2003

Kandyba K, Binik YM: Hypnotherapy as a treatment for vulvar vestibulitis
     syndrome: a case report. J Sex Marital Ther. 29(3): 237–42, 2003

Kaplan HS, Fyer AJ, Novick A: The treatment of sexual phobias: the combined
     use of antipanic medication and sex therapy. J Sex Marital Ther 8:3–28,
     1982

Lamont JA: Female dyspareunia. Am J Obstet Gynecol. 136(3): 282–5, 1980

Marinoff SC, Turner ML: Vulvar vestibulitis syndrome: an overview. Am J
     Obstet Gynecol 165:1228–1233, 1991

Metz ME, Epstein N: Assessing the role of relationship conflict in sexual
     dysfunction. J Sex Marital Ther. 28(2): 139–64, 2002

Mikhail AR: Treatment of vaginismus by i.v. diazepam (Valium) abreaction
     interviews. Acta Psychiatr Scand. 53(5): 328–32, 1976

Montford H: Pelvic pain and dyspareunia. In Rosemarie Lincolin (Eds)
     Psychosexual Medicine. London, Chapman and Hall Publishing
     Company, Inc, pp149–159, 1992

Nappi RE, Ferdeghini F, Abbiati I, et al.: Electrical stimulation (ES) in the
     management of sexual pain disorders. J Sex Marital Ther. 29 Suppl
     1:103–10, 2003

Neidigh L, Kinder BN: The use of audiovisual materials in sex therapy: a critical
     overview. J Sex Marital Ther. 13(1): 64–72, 1987

O'Sullivan K: Observations on vaginismus in Irish women. Arch Gen Psychiatry 36(7): 824–6, 1979

Reissing ED, Binik YM, Khalife S, Cohen D, Amsel R: Etiological correlates of vaginismus: sexual and physical abuse, sexual knowledge, sexual self-schema, and relationship adjustment. J Sex Marital Ther. 29(1): 47–59, 2003

Reissing ED, Binik YM, Khalife S, et al.: Vaginal spasm, pain, and behavior: an empirical investigation of the diagnosis of vaginismus. Arch Sex Behav. 33(1): 5–17, 2004

Reissing ED, Binik YM, Khalife S: Does vaginismus exist? A critical review of the literature. J Nerv Ment Dis. 187(5): 261–74, 1999

Russell L: Sex and couples therapy: a method of treatment to enhance physical and emotional intimacy. J Sex Marital Ther. 16(2): 111–20, 1990

Sandberg G, Quevillon RP: Dyspareunia: an integrated approach to assessment and diagnosis. J Fam Pract. 24(1): 66–70, 1987

Sarazin SK, Seymour SF: Causes and treatment options for women with dyspareunia. Nurse Pract. 16(10): 30, 35–8, 41, 1991

Schnyder U, Schnyder-Luthi C, Ballinari P, Blaser A: Therapy for vaginismus: in vivo versus in vitro desensitization. Can J Psychiatry 43(9): 941–4, 1998

Scholl GM: Prognostic variables in treating vaginismus. Obstet Gynecol. 72(2): 231–5, 1988

Shafik A, El-Sibai O: Study of the pelvic floor muscles in vaginismus: a concept of pathogenesis. Eur J Obstet Gynecol Reprod Biol. 105(1):67–70, 2002

Shaw J: Treatment of primary vaginismus: a new perspective. J Sex Marital Ther. 20(1): 46–55, 1994

Silverstein JL: Origins of psychogenic vaginismus. Psychother Psychosom. 52(4): 197–204, 1989

Simon W, Gagnon JH: Sexual scripts: permanence and change. Arch Sex Behav. 15(2): 97–120, 1986

Spector IP, Carey MP: Incidence and prevalence of the sexual dysfunctions: a critical review of the empirical literature. Arch Sex Behav 19:389–408, 1990

Steege JF, Ling FW: Dyspareunia. A special type of chronic pelvic pain. Obstet Gynecol Clin North Am. 20(4): 779–93, 1993

Steege JF: Dyspareunia and vaginismus Clin Obstet Gynecol. 27(3): 750–9, 1984 van der Velde J, Everaerd W: Voluntary control over pelvic floor muscles in women with and without vaginistic reactions. Int Urogynecol J Pelvic Floor Dysfunct. 10(4): 230–6, 1999

van der Velde J, Laan E, Everaerd W: Vaginismus, a component of a general defensive reaction. an investigation of pelvic floor muscle activity during exposure to emotion-inducing film excerpts in women with and without vaginismus. Int Urogynecol J Pelvic Floor Dysfunct.12(5):328–31, 2001

van Lankveld JJ, Brewaeys AM, Ter Kuile MM, Weijenborg PT: Difficulties in the differential diagnosis of vaginismus, dyspareunia and mixed sexual pain disorder. J Psychosom Obstet Gynaecol. 16(4): 201–9, 1995

van Lankveld JJ: Bibliotherapy in the treatment of sexual dysfunctions: a meta-analysis. J Consult Clin Psychol. Aug; 66(4): 702–8, 1998

Walker E, Katon W, Harrop-Griffiths J, et al: Relationship of chronic pelvic pain to psychiatric diagnoses and childhood sexual abuse. American Journal of Psychiatry 145:75–80, 1988

Walsh KE, Berman JR, Berman LA, Vierregger K: Safety and efficacy of topical nitroglycerin for treatment of vulvar pain in women with vulvodynia: a pilot study. Journal of Gender-Specific Medicine 5(4):21–7, 2002

Walton B, Thorton T: Female sexual dysfunction. Curr Womens Health Rep. Aug;3(4):319–26, 2003

Zimmer D: Does marital therapy enhance the effectiveness of treatment for sexual dysfunction? J Sex Marital Ther. 13(3): 193–209, 1987

# 9

# Alternative Medicine in Sexual Performance Enhancement

LUCY POSTOLOV, L.AC.

## I. Introduction

Cultures around the world have been practicing what Western medicine calls Alternative for over 5000 years. Traditional Oriental Medicine, Homeopathy, Ayurvedic Medicine, Aromatherapy and Meditation, Massages etc. have long been practiced in China, India and the European Continent. These treatments and techniques has been the mainstay of health in these cultures. Although these traditional medical beliefs differ in language, philosophy and metaphors they base their faith on the principle that health is a state of balance or wholeness regulated by a universal life force. This life force is constant with cultures throughout the world. It is called 'qi' (pronounced chi) in China; 'ki' in Japan, 'prana' in India, and the ancient Greeks would know it as 'pneuma'. Medical cultures outside of

Western medicine believe any illness results within the body from unbalances that block the aforementioned life force from flowing freely.

The patient interest in alternative medicines in the 1990's grew at a remarkable rate and continues to gain wider interest and recognition. A report from the National Ambulatory Medical Care Survey conducted in 1990 and 1996, released these remarkable numbers (Ernst 2001). In 1997, visits to all primary care practitioners were 385 million; almost 2 million less than comparable visits in 1990. Conversely, visits to practitioners of alternative therapies rose dramatically from 427 million in 1990 to 628 million in 1997. It would benefit Western medical practitioners greatly to familiarize themselves with the different modalities available to patients and to be well versed in the underlying principles of those medicines (The Burton Goldberg Group 1994).

The patient who has an interest in the some of the techniques mentioned in this chapter, such as Acupuncture, Homeopathy, Ayurveda and Herbal Medicine must seek a licensed or certified practitioner of these arts. In the United States, Acupuncture is a licensed practice in most states. Homeopathy, Ayurveda and Aromatherapy are not licensed, but are certified by credible schools throughout the country. Although they are considered natural healing remedies, they are not to be practiced by the patient on their own.

Western medical science focuses on human sexuality in terms of anatomy, physiology and psychology. In Eastern cultures, sex is regarded as an art, science, and a path to a spiritual development, a path towards greater intimacy not only with the partner but also with the Divine Self.

> Those who understand the nature of sex will nurture their vigor and prolong their life. Those who treat its principle with contempt will injure their spirit and shorten their life.
> —Tung Hsuan Tzu

The most extensive approaches to sex are those of China (Taoism), India (yoga) and Tibet (tantra) which have drawn upon unique ancient classical texts on sexual practices. These texts include: Kama Sutra-Vatsyayana (400 A.D.), Ananga Ranga, Perfumed Garden (fifteenth century), Tao Te Ching-Lao Tzu, (fifth century B.C.), The Yellow Emperor Classics-Huang Ti (2697–2598 B.C.), The Secret Art of Bedchamber (590–618 A.D.), Pillow

Book and the Tantric Buddhism (eigth century). In the Han dynasty there were over 165 books on sexual techniques and 8 different schools on the subject (Beurdeley 1969; Douglas and Slinger 1990; Dunas and Goldberg 1997; Hooper 1994; Maciocia 1998; and Novey 2000).

> Eastern metaphysical traditions make use of the mystery of sexuality as a means to the transcendental experience of unity. The feeling of oneness, achieved during or following the sexual act, is the most universally accessible mystical experience.
> —DOUGLAS AND SLINGER 1979

## II. Traditional Oriental Medicine

A comprehensive system of modalities includes Herbal Medicine, Acupuncture, Massage, Meditation and Exercise.

Chinese philosophers and healers have studied and practiced human sexuality to enhance relationships, vitality, and restore health of the body, mind and spirit. It is very important to note that this philosophy confirms not only an anatomical or physiological difference between man and woman, but also an energetic one.

The feminine energy or 'Yin' is always receiving or "being and opening" the energy of the spirit. The male energy, or 'Yang', is the proactive of the two and is giving and doing. With this responsibility, the man is required to perfect his power of retention. The sexual energy of man is like a fire, quick to get hot, quick to boil, ultimately to explode. The female sexual energy, like water, heats up and boils slowly but staying warm longer.

The Chinese texts 'Classics of the Plain Girl' and 'Counsels of a Simple Girl' are conversations between the legendary Yellow Emperor and his female advisor, Su Nu. She shares with the Emperor the secret methods of lovemaking called the 'Sex Recipes of the Plain Girl' and therapeutic lovemaking, called the 'Discourse of the Plain Girl'. In these books, the Plain Girl declares that "Woman is superior to man in the way that water is superior to fire. People who are experts in the art of love are like excellent cooks who know how to blend the different flavors with a tasty meal. Those who know the art of Yin and Yang can blend the pleasures of the senses, but those who do not know it will have an unexpected death, without ever having enjoyed the art of lovemaking."

The human body has the innate ability to heal itself. It is just a matter of triggering the right mechanisms. Specific points of the body, different breathing techniques and unique postures, channel energy to create balance. Therapeutic lovemaking allows energy to flow freely within the body. Using specific positions in lovemaking helps the energy to be concentrated in specific organs, and at orgasm, the energy is released in this healing way. By using these unique positions, sexual performance will be enhanced and more satisfying to both partners. Sexual problems as well as other health-related issues can also be resolved.

## III. Sexual Positions; Therapeutic Lovemaking

When referring to the ancient texts you will find that many sexual positions are named after animals. Taoist masters believed that by imitating the movements of the animals, humans would be more in tune with nature and bring balance to heaven and earth. Here are just a few of the many positions as described in classical texts.

### A. Mandarin Duck

This position is beneficial for man who has problems sustaining erection and has difficulties with sexual performance. This also improves the concentration of the man's semen. For the woman this position benefits her sexual organs, uterus and ovaries. The position can relieve the symptoms of Premenstrual Syndrome. From the Chinese Medicine point of view it benefits the woman's Yin and strengthens the Jing (essence) of the man.

### B. Pawing Horse

A position that is especially beneficial to the woman who has emotional blockage, mood swings and inability to reach orgasm. The stretch in the pelvic area allows the release of liver energy at the time of orgasm. Her hand is in the 'Mudra' position, known to be beneficial in the release of negative emotions. From the Chinese Medicine view, this position is of benefit for liver qi stagnation.

### C. Overlapping Fish Scale

This position is beneficial to the woman with premenstrual syndrome, fibroid tumors and to regulate menstruation. For the man it can prevent premature ejaculation and low back pain. The Chinese medical benefits are; tonifys blood in liver channel for woman and for man tonifys kidney yin deficiency.

### D. Tiger Attacks

Improves the immune system and bone marrow production. Also helps pain in the spine for woman. A position that is beneficial for harmonizing life force (Qi) and balances all five elements.

### E. Crane with Two Necks

A position that creates and sustains a harmonious sexual relationship. The couple is seated in close union and learns to give as well as receive sexual energy. From the Chinese medicine point of view, benefits 'Three Treasures' being Shen 'spirit', Qi 'energy' and Jing 'essence'.

### F. Flattering Phoenix

This position is tranquilizing the life force. Helps the woman with PMS and fibroids and harmonizes the joints of the man. From the Chinese medicine point of view beneficial for woman with blood Qi stagnation and man with kidney deficiency.

## IV. Description of Acupuncture and Chinese Herbal Medicine

### A. Acupuncture

A treatment that involves puncturing the skin with hair-thin needles inserted into underlying tissue. The word acupuncture originated from the Latin 'acus' (needle) and 'puncture' (puncture) and originated in China some 5000 years ago. A typical treatment consists of needles inserted at specific points in the body, extremities, face and ears along lines called meridians and channels. These meridians and channels are vessels for the life force or 'Qi' to flow freely. Through diagnosis unique to the Chinese Medicine Practitioner, observation of the tongue, palpation of abdomen and meridians, and traditional pulse palpation, it is determined where blockages, stagnation or deficiency of energy occurs. One of the essential aspects of Chinese diagnosis is based on the Five Elements theory. Each element: Fire, Earth, Metal, Water and Wood have corresponding organs, channels and emotions. When out of balance, the problem manifests.

| | Organ | Emotion | Archtype | Sexual Values | Desire | Addition to be | Fear to be |
|---|---|---|---|---|---|---|---|
| **Fire** | Heart/ Small Intestine | Joy | Wizard | Orgasm Merging | Fulfillment | In Love | Cut off |
| **Earth** | Spleen Stomach | Overthinking/ Worry | Peacemaker | Embracing Connectedness | Connectedness | Needed | Lost |
| **Metal** | Lung/Large Intestine | Grief/Sadness | Alchemist | Sacred Ritual Ceremony | Order | Right | Corrupted |
| **Water** | Kidney/Urinary Bladder | Fear Fright | Philosopher | Penetration/ Mystery | Truth | Protected | Extinct |
| **Wood** | Liver/ Gallbladder | Anger | Pioneer | More, Better, Longer | Purpose | Arousal | Helpless |

**TABLE 1**
**Correlation of 5 Elements and Emotions**

In *Acupuncture: Textbook & Atlas*, Stux and Pomeranz (1987) conclude that acupuncture activates small myelineated nerve fibers in the muscle, which send impulses to the spinal cord, and then activates three centers (spinal cord, midbrain, and pituitary-hypothalamus. While in the book *Neuro-Acupuncture*, Cho et al. (2001) write 'Early work on the beta-endorphin theory suggests that there is cortical involvement following acupuncture stimulation. Indeed, a number of acupuncture analgesia theories are successfully explained by some cortical involvement, such as the humoral function of the hypothalamus and the brainstem. It is increasingly clear that acupuncture stimulation leads to activation of the upper parts of the brain or upper cortical areas via various spinal tracts. Many of its collateral's project to the lower parts of the brain, from the upper midbrain to the pons and medulla, where many survival-related autonomic functions are believed to be regulated'.

In Figure 1, conceptual relationship between the brain, organs and acupuncture is illustrated. This illustration is a conceptual

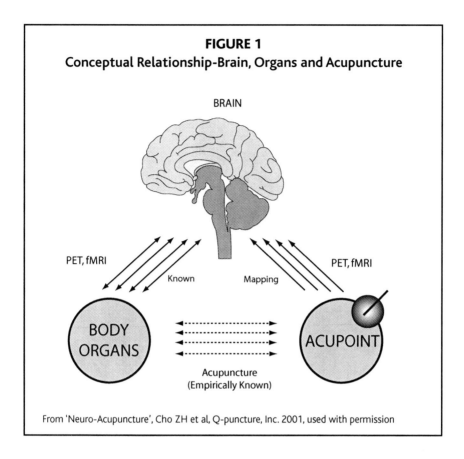

**FIGURE 1**

**Conceptual Relationship-Brain, Organs and Acupuncture**

BRAIN

PET, fMRI

Known     Mapping

PET, fMRI

BODY ORGANS

ACUPOINT

Acupuncture
(Empirically Known)

From 'Neuro-Acupuncture', Cho ZH et al, Q-puncture, Inc. 2001, used with permission

relationship deduced from the correlation study between the treatment effects of diseases stated for each acupoint and their related cortical activation.

In Figure 2, note that pain control is only a small part of the broader survival-related functions of acupuncture disease treatment, including endocrine, autonomic and neurochemical functions. These are mainly controlled by the hypothalamus, the central integrator and controller of the body and the brain (Cho 2001).

### B.  Traditional Chinese Herbal Medicine

One of the most ancient forms of healthcare began with Shen Nong Ben Cao Jing (Pharmacopoeia of the Heavenly Husbandman) in the second century B.C.

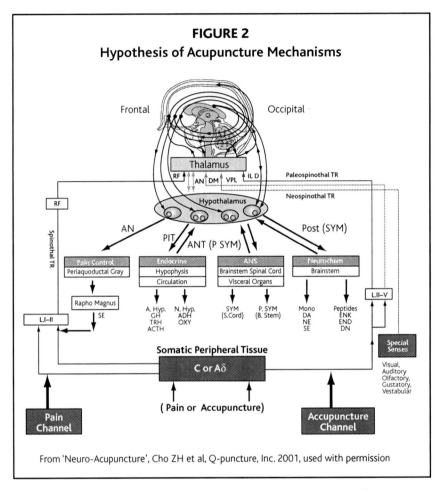

**FIGURE 2**
**Hypothesis of Acupuncture Mechanisms**

From 'Neuro-Acupuncture', Cho ZH et al, Q-puncture, Inc. 2001, used with permission

Chinese herbs are effective when prescribed according with traditional Chinese diagnosis. They work the same way, as do conventional pharmaceutical drugs via their chemical reactions.

## V. Exercises and Techniques to Enhance Sexual Performance

### A. Microcosmic Orbits (Chia and Wei, 2003)

With the male's genitals being external and the females internal, the union of the two provides an opportunity for the yin and the yang to mesh and achieve a perfect exchange of energy. Emotionally, the woman is yang energy; it is easier for her to express herself. Physically the woman is yin, while the male is physically yang and emotionally yin. During the act of intercourse, the male, with his external sexual yang energy is the giver to the female's internal sexual yin energy. Emotionally, vice versa, the female gives through her heart and the male receives. Together, they compliment and balance each other's energy, sexually and emotionally.

B. **Kegel Exercise and Its Variation** from Taoist practice for both men and women:

1. Rapid contraction and release of pelvic area for one to two minutes

2. Slow contraction and release of pelvic area for one to two minutes
   A woman can improve her sexual experience by strengthening the muscles in the vaginal wall by inserting two fingers in her vagina during these contractions. Also effective would be the Jade Egg, a more traditional device.

C. **Massage the Ears**
   With the ears each having over 150 acupuncture points, they are an excellent source for stimulation of sexual energy. In Chinese medicine, the ear is an extension of the Kidney energy, which is responsible for sexuality. A couple instinctively massages, kisses and nibbles each other's ears during lovemaking. When the ear is massaged, it stimulates the entire body (Oleson 1996).

D. **Taoist Retention of the Semen Exercise**
   The Taoist man uses his mind to control his breath, his breath to control his blood, and his blood to control the semen. By mastering breathing techniques and utilizing them during lovemaking, the male can control his heartbeat, which speeds up before ejaculation. Using deep, rhythmic abdominal breathing, he is able to control his heartbeat and thus 'quiet' the rush of blood to the penis, suppressing the ejaculation.

   Of all the things that make mankind prosper, none can be compared to sexual intercourse. It is modeled after Heaven and takes its form by Earth; it regulates Yin and rules Yang...Thus the four seasons succeed each other; man thrusts, woman receives; above there is action; below, receptivity.
   —Taoist Master

## VI.  Foods as Aphrodisiacs

The legend and reality of the existence of Aphrodisiacs has been questioned through time. The truth of the matter is that indeed there are foods that are rich in minerals, vitamins and essential fatty acids that in both short and long term can enhance the sexual libido (Nickell 1999).

| | |
|---|---|
| **Foods:** | oysters, shrimp, mustard, garlic, leeks, avocado, nuts, seeds, kelp, yogurt, eggs, beans |
| **Minerals:** | Iodine, Magnesium, Manganese, Zinc, Chromium, and Calcium |
| **Essential Fatty Acids:** | L-Arginine, Phenylalanine and Tyrosine, Phenyletbylamine |
| **Vitamins:** | Vitamin E, $B_1$, $B_2$, $B_3$, $B_6$, $B_{12}$, Folic Acid, and Vitamin C |

All foods, vitamins and minerals should be taken in moderation and not exceed the daily dietary requirements.

## VII. Aromatherapy

A sense that is frequently overlooked, smell plays an important role in our lives. One of the most primal senses, its power has only recently begun to be explored. The sense of smell is unique in that it evades the cerebral cortex. Smell receptors in the nose are directly connected to the limbic center, which controls emotions, moods, memories, and sex drive. It is therefore very common to get a whiff of a familiar scent and be nostalgic of a person, place, and time in ones life without the control of our conscious mind.

Aromatherapy uses the power of plant chemicals as well as other smells to arouse the body, elevate emotions and mood, and create a desired ambiance. Specific smells are often used to increase sex drive and sexual arousal, often unconsciously. Aromas are usually contained in essential oils, and can be used as inhalants or mixed with base oils and used as massage oil; either way serving as an erotic stimulant.

A number of smells are responsible for triggering sexual memories and excitement and are attainable at most health stores. For example: *Ambergris,* a mild, sweet, earthy smelling aroma continues to be used in Asia as an aphrodisiac. Often coffee would be laced with ambergris to exhibit its aphrodisiac quality when taken orally. In the novel Moby Dick, ambergris, was the highly prized, sweet smelling product of a sperm whale; in reality, it is the vomit of a sperm whale caused by digestive irritation. Although the thought of whale vomit may not seem romantic, the smell is very pleasant. Once their rare power were discovered, not only was it distributed as oil, but also perfume manufactures began to incorporate ambergris in fine fragrances, especially those with floral hints.

Both jasmine and rose have intoxicating smells capable of exciting either sex. Fragrances containing jasmine are very expensive because oil extraction is very laborious as well as tedious. Jasmine has the power to strengthen male sex organs, low libido, as well as treat impotence and prostate problems. It has also been used an anti-depressant. The precious fragrance of rose is also esteemed and was once used by kings. If jasmine is the king, rose is its queen. Rose has been the choice in various ceremonies and love potions. It is said that when Cleopatra met Anthony, she layered her floor an inch deep with rose petals an action typical in Rome where rose petals were scattered at weddings as well as bridal beds. Rose oil is also hard to extract and is expensive oil, however highly sought after for several reasons. The smell is very sensual and seemingly popular therefore arousing erotic memories. It is also a mood elevator and may contain phenyl ethanol, which has narcotic properties. The sweet smell of rose, like ylang-ylang, is calming and pacifies anxiety and stress.

Perhaps the most provocative fragrance, musk, has been referred to as the 'universal' aphrodisiac. Derived from the Sanskrit word for testicle, it is a scent produced my males in nature. Nonetheless, this general term for the erosion of male hormones is rousing for both sexes. Musk oil was the preferred fragrance of Josephine Bonaparte, Napoleon's wife, and when he decided to leave her she poured the oil all over the bedroom so he would never forget her. Musk has an unmistaken and obstinate smell. Originally acquired from the abdominal gland from the male musk deer, today it is synthesized as galaxolide and Exaltoilde. Unlike the other smells discussed musk provokes the VNO, a special organ identifying pheromones, because it produces alpha-androstenol. For this reason musk is not only erotic through smell but also a hormone related substance.

Smells from nature have been used to arouse for centuries, but for a long time natural smell was over looked. It is evident that animals are sexually stimulated by smells (dogs in heat), and even recognize territories. Can humans have a similar attraction through smells? The VNO (vomeronasal organ) found in the nostrils, detects pheromones, chemical messengers similar to hormones, among humans. Dr. David Berliner was researching an unrelated topic and was scraping skin cells from used casts of skiers. He made extracts from the cells in vials. Whenever Berliner left the vials open, the atmosphere of the lab was much friendlier. When they were closed the lab chaos resumed. Hearing about the discovery of the VNO, Berliner teemed up with Dr. Luis Monti-Bloch to test the human VNO. After puffing pure air, scented air, Berliner's two compounds, air without hormones or pheromones, and fragrant compound, the two men found that the VNO only reacted to Berliner's extracts. In addition, male subjects reacted to female extract and vice versa. When the men tested the olfactory nerves, the subject only responded to the fragrant smell. This evidence gave rise to more questions and initiated the discovery of pheromones as aphrodisiacs.

Pheromones are produced in sweat glands and appear where hair is highly concentrated. Bacteria are trapped in and as they decompose pheromones are released. The aroma from pheromones is often called a persons smell and is as individual as fingerprints. Males secrete a musky odor, which is paired with the odor-producing skin bacteria. The female pheromones result from estrogen and progesterone, which control the odor men release, and fluctuate during the monthly cycle. While pheromones do not stimulate sexual activity, they arouse an erotic mood. Using synthetic hormones has been reported to make people feel more attractive and romantic. They also explain certain degrees of sexual attraction, when a person cannot understand what they see in someone that may simply be compatible pheromones. Tight clothes restrict the release of pheromones that are natural sex enhancers. The smell of sweat on a lover's body after a workout is very arousing because that same smell is secreted during lovemaking. Couples sleeping on foreign sides of the bed are the VNO recognizing the pheromones that are still lingering, providing comfort.

Different smells will appeal to different people although the ingredients are the same. The chemistry of the smell with the individual will vary.

The power of smell plays a major role in lovemaking and can enhance the arousal and pleasure.

## VIII. Ayurvedic Medicine

### A. Introduction

The origins of Ayurveda can be found in India over five thousand years ago. Ayurvedic (meaning 'science of life') medicine places its emphasis on the state of the individual body, mind and spirit, in equal proportions. As with many Alternative approaches to medicine and health, the prominence of prevention is the approach to a patient's health as opposed to curing a disease.

Upon the patient's initial visit to the Ayurvedic practitioner, the individual constitution is determined by determining the metabolic body type or *doshas*. The practitioner will base the diagnosis on physical observation, personal and family history, palpation and listening to the heart, lungs and intestines. Particular consideration will be paid to the pulse, tongue, eyes and nails. In Ayurveda medicine, the concept of metabolic types is categorized in three distinctive doshas. These doshas are known as *vata*, *pitta*, and *kapha*. The characteristics of these doshas include a number of different factors unique to the individual. Some contributing (but not limited to) features are build, hair, skin, temper, appetite, sleeping habits, energy level, personality, and sexual desire.

Most individuals will have predominance in one of the dosha body types, but all three will be present. Equally, the three doshas are located in specific areas of the body. The individual is at most favorable health when all doshas are in balance.

### B. Sexual Balance

Each dosha has characteristics and responsibilities unique to the development of sexuality. Sexual realization is attained when the correct equilibrium is reached among the doshas.

The dosha *vata* is responsible for the movement of the body. If depleted, there will be an adverse reaction in the actual act of sex and retention of the sexual energy.

*Pitta* is the impetus for sexual drive. When there is an imbalance in the pitta dosha, you will find a lack of initiative in sexual activity. Accompanying this state will be physical manifestations (rashes, herpes outbreaks, acne, odors etc.) that would make this person less desirable for sexual interest.

Finally, *kapha* takes on the responsibility of sexual potency. An imbalance here will directly affect the fertility and effectiveness of the sexual excretions. Finding exhaustion in the kapha will directly affect the ability to procreate.

### C. Treatment Plan

After diagnosis of the disease or the imbalance of the individual, the practitioner has four methods of management available to obtain the desired results; Cleansing and detoxification (*Shodan*), Palliation (*Shaman*), Rejuvenation (*Rasayana*) and Mental Hygiene (*Satvajaya*).

### D. Improving Sexual Performance with Ayurvedic Medicine

The Ayurvedic practitioner will address the individual's sexual concerns after a systematic management plan is in place to balance the doshas. After the patient has been cleansed and detoxed, the practitioner will look to rejuvenate and enhance the body's ability to function. Herbs are commonly used to address sexual problems and to enhance the sexual abilities of the individual. Here are two recipes that may be used for specific sexual purpose (Vinod 1997):

1. Premature Ejaculation: Put a pinch of camphor in ⅛ cup (25ml) Rose essence and mix well. Apply this on the penis in a very small quantity by putting 2–3 drops of it on your fingers and then smearing it on penis about an hour before intercourse.

2. Increase desire: This is a very simple preparation with readily available ingredients. You need powdered licorice, ghee, honey and milk. For one dose, mix 1 tablespoon each: powdered licorice, honey and ghee. Whip well. You should obtain a kind of paste that should be eaten with some hot milk. It is excellent to increase the sexual urge.

Ayurveda medicine, as many of the 'Alternative' medicines, has been practiced and utilized by patients around the world for thousands of years. Its popularity and success rate in India and Europe cannot be ignored. As the demand for this technique in the Western countries continues to rise, research that is more clinical will be conducted and given credence.

## IX. Homeopathy

### A. Introduction

Homeopathy is a form of holistic medicine based on Hippocrates Law of Similars (Like cures like) with the premise that "through the like, disease is produced, and through the application of the like, it is cured." In order for a homeopathic treatment to cure a disease, it must produce similar symptoms of the disease in a healthy person. This of course is a principle that is the theoretical basis for the vaccines of Edward Jenner, Jonas Salk, and Louis Pasteur. A practice founded in the late eighteenth century by German physician, Samuel Hahnemann (2002), the word homeopathy is derived from the Greek word "homois" meaning similar and "pathos" meaning disease. Hahnemann was translating medical text when he learned about *cinchona*, a Peruvian bark that was used in the treatment of malaria. Hahnemann experimented with the substance and ingested it twice daily. Upon taking his own mixture with Peruvian bark, he began to develop symptoms similar to malaria. The same substance, when taken in a smaller, regulated dose would stimulate the body to fight the disease. Hahnemann went on to test hundreds of plants, minerals, and animals to discover that many of these produced symptoms similar to the disease that they cured. It is here that Hahnemann formulated the principles of homeopathy.

In addition to the *Law of Similars*, Homeopathy is also based on the *Law of the Infinitesimal Dose*. The more a remedy is diluted, the more potent its strength in fighting the disease. Typically, a single dose of a homeopathic substance would be 10 drops placed below a 'clean' tongue. More is not better, and when an additional dose is taken, it will interfere with the action of the first dose and harm the balance being created. One dose on the other hand will catalyze the body to make a change. Unlike Western medicine, where a higher dosage means increased strength, homeopathy requires the lowest possible dose to stimulate the body's own healing powers. With the effect being similar to an enzyme or a hormone, a small amount results in a large change. In addition, Hahnemann was concerned by the side effects of frequently used medications and found that medications that were diluted reduced side effects and maintained effectiveness. Striking and shaking the homeopathic solution increased the substance's medicinal properties, conveying that diluted and whisked treatments had stronger medicinal effects (Merani 1994).

There are specific substances, plant, mineral and animal, which have a history of being effective with sexual enhancement and certain dysfunctions. With the proper guidance of a Homeopath, remedies can be both safe and effective. The practice of homeopathy works with an individuals self-healing powers. An alternative form of medicine, homeopathy focuses on energy or "chi" and seeing how an individual's body works as a whole. Hahnemann explained that treatments create a stronger force that overpowers the illness and produces a cure. Homeopathy also uses water's power as a solvent to carry information about its solute and become more potent with repeated usage and addition of solute.

The FDA (Food and Drug Administration) recognizes homeopathic remedies as official drugs and regulates the manufacture, labeling and dispensing. The remedies have their own official compendium, the Homeopathic Pharmacopoeia of the United States that was first published in 1897.

Homeopathy is a low cost, safe system of medicine that should be explored further. Millions of people around the world are already using homeopathic remedies effectively and in a self care environment.


## X. Conclusion and Future Directions

Alternative medicine strategies of sexual enhancement are gaining a more important role in Sexual Medicine especially that they are gaining public interest and approval. More studies showing empirical evidence of these strategies are underway.

# *References*

Beurdeley M et al., Chinese Erotic Art. VT: Charles E. Tuttle Company Inc., 1969

Chia M and Wei WU: Sexual Reflexology. VT: Destiny Books, 2003

Cho ZH et al., Neuro-Acupuncture. Los Angeles, CA: Q-puncture, Inc., 2001

Douglas N and Slinger P, Sexual Secrets. VT: Destiny Books, 1979

Douglas N and Slinger P, The Erotic Sentiment in the Paintings of China & Japan. VT: Park Street Press, 1990

Dunas F and Goldberg P, Passion Play. New York, NY: Riverhead, 1997

Ernst E, The Desktop Guide to Complimentary and Alternative Medicine. London, UK: Harcourt Publishers Limited, 2001

Hahnemann S and Boericke W, Organon of Medicine, New Translated Ed. New Delhi: B. Jain Publishers Pvt. Ltd., 2002

Hooper A, Kamasutra. NY: Dorling Kindersley Publishing, Inc., 1994

Maciocia, G: Obstetrics & Gynecology in Chinese Medicine. NY: Churchill Livingstone, 1998

Merani VH, The Practitioner's Hand Book of Homoeopathy. New Delhi: B. Jain Publishers Pvt. Ltd., 1994

Nickell N, Nature's Aphrodisiacs. CA: Crossing Press, Inc., 1999

Novey DW, Complementary & Alternative Medicine. Missouri: Mosby, Inc., 2000

Oleson T, Auriculotherapy Manual. Los Angeles, CA: Health Care Alternatives, Inc., 1996

Stux G and Pomeranz B, Acupuncture: textbook and atlas. Berlin: Springer-Verlag, 1987

The Burton Goldberg Group, Alternative Medicine. WA: Future Medicine Publishing, 1994

Vinod V, Ayurveda for Life.: Nutrition, Sexual Energy & Healing. ME: Samuel Weiser, Inc., 1997

# 10

# Women's Sexual Health

LAURA A.C. BERMAN, LCSW, PHD
ELIZABETH L. WOOD, LSW
DEE HARTMANN, PT

## I. Introduction

From the few studies that have addressed the treatment of sexual complaints in a medical setting, one study revealed that 70 percent of patients said they would consult a family physician for a sexual problem. Family physicians were chosen more frequently than gynecologists, friends, therapists or clergy (Liese et al. 1987). In one web-based survey, 4,000 women with sexual dysfunction were asked about their experiences seeking help from their health care professionals (Berman et al. 2003). Only 40% of the women reported that they did not seek help from a physician for sexual function complaints, but 54% of those reported that they would have liked to but did not for such reasons as embarrassment, believing the physician wouldn't be able to help, or simply that they weren't asked about their sexual functioning.

There are many reasons why a healthcare professional may not will-ingly deal with a patient's sexual concerns. In an older population of patients, physicians may subscribe to larger social norms that devalue sexu-ality among the aged, viewing them as asexual or not capable of sustaining a sexual relationship. In more general terms, the physician may experi-ence anxiety when confronting his or her own unresolved sexual issues or conflicts in the face of the patients' complaints. Finally, medicine is only just beginning to address female sexual function complaints and obtain an adequate scientific knowledge base in order to effectively treat these prob-lems; certainly, this lack of understanding and knowledge may be a factor in many doctors' unwillingness to deal with sexual issues.

Many clinicians believe that the occurrence of sexual concerns is rare in their practice. It seems likely that this is the result of a self-fulfilling prophecy. The patients identify their sexual problem as a physical problem best dealt with by a physician, but they expect the physician to initiate the discussion as he or she would with regard to other functional systems (Metz et al. 1993). If questions of sexual functioning are not included in a systems review, the patient and physician miss an opportunity to connect on this dimension of her life.

The prevalence of female sexual dysfunction is a topic that has gen-erated extensive discussion in both the medical and lay communities alike. According to the National Health and Social Life Survey, approxi-mately 43 percent of American women suffer from sexual dysfunction (Laumann et al. 1999). U.S. population census data reveal that 9.7 million American women ages 50–74 self-report complaints of decreased arousal, diminished vaginal lubrication, pain and discomfort with intercourse, and difficulty achieving orgasm. Female sexual dysfunction is clearly an important woman's health issue that affects the quality of life of many female patients.

With this high prevalence of sexual concerns in the population, women are likely to identify their physician as the professional most frequently consulted about sexual concerns. Furthermore, they expect their doctor to take a leadership role in raising the issue of sexual health. They expect empathy, warmth, confidentiality, and professional competence in discuss-ing their sexual concerns with their physician.

## II. Overview of Sexual Complaints

Sexual complaints in women, known as female sexual dysfunction (FSD) has historically been considered a problem rooted in psychology. However, while there are emotional and relationship elements to sexual function, it has become increasingly evident that female sexual dysfunction can have organic roots and occur secondary to medical problems. Ongoing epidemiological studies in women suggest that the same disease processes and risk factors that are associated with male erectile dysfunction including aging, hypertension, cigarette smoking and hypercholesterolemia are also associated with female sexual dysfunction (Hsueh et al. 1998).

However, in order to understand the etiologies and treatments, it is important to first understand the physiology of the sexual response cycle, more details are provided in Chapter 1 on the Sexual Response Cycle. The successive phases of sexual response include arousal (otherwise considered excitement and plateau phases), orgasm, and resolution (Masters et al. 1966). During sexual arousal, both the clitoris and the labia minora become engorged with blood, and vaginal and clitoral length and diameter both increase. The labia minora also increase in diameter by two to three times during sexual excitement and consequently become everted, exposing their inner surface. The component of 'desire' as preceding and inciting the entire sexual response cycle was first proposed by Helen Singer Kaplan (Kaplan 1966). Kaplan's three-phase model of desire, orgasm, and resolution is the basis for the DSM IV definitions of female sexual dysfunction, as well as the recent re-classification system made by the American Foundation of Urologic Disease (AFUD) Consensus Panel in October of 1998 (Basson et al. 2000). Others have recently suggested that sexual function should be considered as a circuit, with four main domains: libido, arousal, orgasm, and satisfaction. Each aspect may overlap and/or negatively or positively affect the next (Graziottin 1996).

## AFUD Classification and Definition of Female Sexual Disorders

The American Foundation of Urologic Disease (AFUD) consensus panel included 19 experts in female sexual dysfunction selected from 5 countries. This interdisciplinary team brought together specialists from the fields of endocrinology, family medicine, gynecology, nursing, pharmacology, physiology, psychiatry, psychology, rehabilitation medicine, and urology. The objective of the panel was to evaluate and revise existing definitions and classifications of female sexual dysfunction so that they would cross disciplines. Specifically, medical risk factors and etiologies for female sexual dysfunction were incorporated with the pre-existing psychologically based definitions. The following classifications are sub-typed as lifelong versus acquired, generalized versus situational, and organic versus psychogenic or mixed. Most importantly, in order for a woman to be diagnosed with FSD, she must be experiencing significant personal distress. The etiology of any of these disorders may be multi-factorial, and often times the disorders overlap (Basson et al. 2000).

### A. Hypoactive Sexual Desire Disorder (HSDD)

HSDD is defined as the persistent or recurring deficiency (or absence) of sexual fantasies, thoughts, and/or receptivity to sexual activity, which causes personal distress. Sexual Aversion Disorder is used to describe a persistent or recurring phobic aversion to and active avoidance of sexual contact.

Hypoactive sexual desire disorder may have physiologic roots, such as hormone deficiencies, or may result from medical or surgical interventions. Any disruption of the female hormonal milieu caused by natural menopause, surgically or medically induced menopause, or endocrine disorders, can result in inhibited sexual desire. Furthermore, the lack of desire may actually be secondary to poor arousal, response or pain. More details on Sexual Desire Disorders are provided in Chapter 5.

### B. Female Sexual Arousal Disorder (FSAD)

FSAD is the persistent or recurring inability to attain or maintain adequate sexual excitement, causing personal distress. It may be experienced as a lack of subjective excitement or a lack of genital (lubrication/swelling) or other somatic responses. Disorders of arousal include, but are not limited to, lack of or diminished vaginal lubrication, decreased clitoral and labial sensation, decreased clitoral and labial engorgement, or lack of vaginal smooth muscle relaxation. There may be a medical/physiologic basis for FSAD such as diminished vaginal/clitoral blood flow, prior pelvic trauma, pelvic surgery, or medications. More details on Sexual Arousal Disorders are provided in Chapter 6.

## C. Female Orgasmic Disorder (FOD)

FOD is the persistent or recurrent difficulty, delay in, or absence of attaining orgasm, following sufficient sexual stimulation and arousal that causes personal distress. FOD may be a primary anorgasmia (never achieved orgasm) or a secondary anorgasmic condition (was able to achieve orgasm at one point in time, but now no longer able). FOD can even be situational, referring to the woman who can experience orgasm in some circumstances (e.g. masturbation), but cannot in other situations.

Another kind of anorgasmia commonly experienced by women is Coital FOD, or the inability to achieve orgasm from coital thrusting without added sexual stimulation. Only 30% of women experience orgasm regularly from sexual intercourse, 30% never reach orgasm during intercourse, and 40% have difficulty achieving orgasm from coital thrusting alone (Lamont 1994). Many women describing themselves as anorgasmic are in fact experiencing coital anorgasmia.

Secondary FOD is often a result of surgery, trauma, or hormone deficiencies. Primary FOD is typically secondary to emotional trauma or sexual abuse, and Situational FOD, while often also associated with a trauma history, is also commonly related to emotional stressors and relationship conflicts. However, in both of these cases medical/physical factors, as well as medications (i.e. selective serotonin re-uptake inhibitors), can contribute to or exacerbate the problem. More details on Orgasmic Disorders are provided in Chapter 7.

## D. Sexual Pain Disorders

### 1. Chronic Vulvar Pain

The etiology of chronic vulvar pain is varied, with a number of diagnoses leading to multiple symptoms. Among disorders causing vulvar pain are vulvodynia; cyclic vulvovaginitis; pudendal neuralgia; contact and inflammatory dermatitis; previous obstetric or gynecologic trauma to the vagina; menopausal or radiation atrophy; inflammation of the urinary tract, rectum, or vagina; or fixation of pelvic tissues. Chronic constipation can also be a primary source of discomfort. The chronic complex can be either physiological or psychological or a combination of the two (Lamont 1990; Lamont 1980).

Vulvodynia is defined as vulvar discomfort; most often described as burning pain, occurring in the absence of relevant visible findings or of a specific, clinically identifiable, neurologic disorder. It can be classified as "local" or "generalized" and as "provoked" or "unprovoked" (Haefner et al. 2004). Approximately 16% of women questioned in a recent study reported complaints of chronic burning, knifelike pain, or pain with contact on the vulva that has lasted for longer than 3 months. Nearly 40% of the women with pain chose not to seek medical care, and of those who did seek treatment, 60% had seen 3 or more doctors, many of whom could not diagnose the problem (Harlow et al. 2003). Cyclic vulvovaginitis (CVV) causes pain just prior to a woman's menstrual cycle. With the etiology multifactorial, CVV often results from hypersensitivity to *Candida Albicans*, changes in the acidity of the vagina (pH), and/or selective IgA deficiency. Vulvar dysesthesias frequently are a result of pudendal neuralgia, a neurological disorder of the pudendal nerve, which serves the lower pelvis. Contact vulvar dermatosis can bring about an acute, noncyclic vulvar discharge, which results in a burning type pain in women who are typically peri- or post-menopausal (Walsh et al. 2002; McKay 1988).

## 2. Dyspareunia

Dyspareunia is a chronic and recurrent genital pain that occurs with intercourse. It, too, is multifactorial, with possible medical and/or psychological origins. Medical conditions that can cause painful intercourse include recurrent vaginal infections, menopausal changes in the vaginal tissue (thinning, dryness), and post-surgical complications. Psychological issues such as emotional or relationship conflicts can also lead to dyspareunia (Berman et al. 2001). Pain with intercourse can also be a result of a change in the physiologic sexual response or arousal phase (vaginal lubrication and expansion and pelvic floor muscle relaxation), which promotes comfortable intercourse.

### 3. Vaginismus

Vaginismus, an involuntary spasm of the vaginal wall with attempted vaginal entry, is another sexual pain disorder that involves both physical and psychological etiologies. Though historically referred to as purely a disorder of fear, guilt, or dissatisfaction (Bengston 1995), physical factors, such as endometriosis and recurrent vaginal or urinary tract infections, can also play an active role in sustaining symptoms (Berman et al. 1998).

More details on Sexual Pain Disorders are provided in Chapter 8.

## III. General Etiologies of Female Sexual Dysfunction

### A. Vasculogenic

Sexual dysfunction in women and impotence in men have been associated with high blood pressure, high cholesterol levels, smoking, and heart disease. The recently named clitoral and vaginal vascular insufficiency syndromes are, in fact, directly related to diminished genital blood flow, secondary to atherosclerosis of the iliohypogastric/pudendal arterial bed (Goldstein et al. 1999). Although other underlying conditions, either psychological or physiological/organic, may also manifest as decreased vaginal and clitoral engorgement, arterial insufficiency is one etiology that should be considered.

Diminished pelvic blood flow secondary to aortoiliac or atherosclerotic disease leads to vaginal wall and clitoral smooth muscle fibrosis. This ultimately results in symptoms of vaginal dryness and dyspareunia. While the precise mechanism is not known, it is possible that the atherosclerotic changes that occur in clitoral vascular and trabecular smooth muscle interfere with normal relaxation and dilation responses to sexual simulation.

Aside from atherosclerotic disease, alterations in circulating estrogen levels associated with menopause contribute to the age-associated changes in clitoral and vaginal smooth muscle. Additionally, any traumatic injury to the iliohypogastric/pudendal arterial bed from pelvic fractures, blunt trauma, surgical disruption, or chronic perineal pressure from bicycle riding, for instance, can result in diminished vaginal and clitoral blood flow and complaints of sexual dysfunction.

### B.  Musculogenic

The muscles of the pelvic floor are invested in female sexual responsiveness as well as in sexual function. A duo of small superficial muscles (bulbocavernosus and ischicavernosus) encircles the vagina and is responsible for the involuntary rhythmic contractions during orgasm. When exercised regularly, they can intensify and contribute to arousal and orgasm. In addition, the muscles of the deep pelvic floor (pubococcygeus or PC) also modulate motor responses vaginal receptivity during orgasm. Hypertonicity within these two groups can lead to sexual dysfunction and pain disorders.

### C. Neurogenic

The same neurogenic etiologies that cause erectile dysfunction in men can also cause sexual dysfunction in women. These include: 1) spinal cord injury or disease of the central or peripheral nervous system, including diabetes and 2) complete upper motor neuron injuries affecting sacral spinal segments. Women with incomplete injuries may retain that capacity for psychogenic arousal and vaginal lubrication (Goldstein et al.1998). With regard to orgasm, women with spinal cord injury have significantly more difficulty achieving orgasm than normal controls (Sipski et al. 1995). The effects of specific spinal cord injuries on female sexual response as well as the role for vasoactive pharmacotherapy in this population are being investigated.

### D.  Hormonal/Endocrine

Dysfunction of the hypothalamic/pituitary axis, hypopituitarism, Addison's disease, corticosteroid therapy, ovarian failure or oophorectomy, menopause, oral estrogen replacement therapy or oral contraceptive use, and surgical removal of the gonads are the most common causes of hormonally based female sexual dysfunction. The most common complaints associated with decreased estrogen and/or testosterone levels are decreased libido, vaginal dryness, and lack of sexual arousal. While testosterone replacement is not FDA approved for use in women, more research is being done every day to determine the causes of androgen deficiency in women and the most effective ways to replace it. Protocols for replacing testosterone will be addressed in the treatment section.

Although estrogen replacement therapy comes with its own host of risks, we know that estrogen improves the integrity of vaginal mucosal tissue and has beneficial effects on vaginal sensation, vasocongestion, and secretions, which all leads to enhanced arousal. Estrogen deprivation causes a significant decrease in clitoral intracavenosal blood flow and vaginal and urethral blood flow. Histologically, it causes diffuse clitoral fibrosis, thinned vaginal epithelial layers, and decreased vaginal submucosal vasculature. Thus, a decline in circulating estrogen levels can produce significant adverse effects on structure and function of the vagina and clitoris, ultimately affecting sexual function.

### E. Psychosocial Factors

It is important to remember that in women, despite the presence or absence of organic disease, emotional and relationship issues significantly affect sexual function and response. In every woman with a sexual function complaint, there are relationship, emotional, and medical factors happening simultaneously and interacting with one another in a non-linear fashion. From the relationship standpoint (**See Table 1**), partner sexual dysfunction, uneven levels of desire, lack of communication, relationship conflict, lack of information about sexual stimulation, and how each defines sexual satisfaction/gratification can all impact on a woman's sexual response.

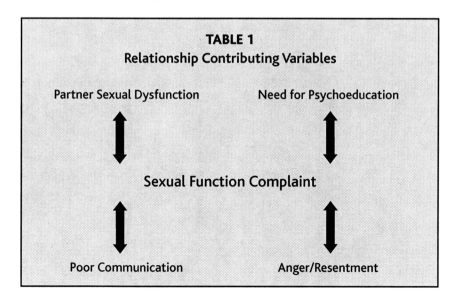

**TABLE 1**
**Relationship Contributing Variables**

Partner Sexual Dysfunction     Need for Psychoeducation

**Sexual Function Complaint**

Poor Communication     Anger/Resentment

For instance, the majority of heterosexual women and their partners believe that they should be able to obtain orgasm through sexual intercourse. Failure to achieve this goal can result in sexual dissatisfaction, relationship conflict, and a lack of sexual confidence. It is important to remember that when a woman struggles with a sexual function complaint, it may create conflict in the relationship, which then cycles back to negatively affect her function.

The same is true for the emotional part of the equation (see **Table 2**). For the woman herself, issues such as self-esteem and body image, a history of sexual trauma or emotional abuse, drug and/or alcohol abuse and sexual addiction can affect her ability to respond sexually. An inability to respond sexually is often connected to performance anxiety. The first time she is unable to respond, it may be situational or circumstantial, but because every time she is sexual after that she worries it might happen again, her response may be inhibited.

Other mood disorders and psychological stressors like depression; anxiety, chronic stress and fatigue are all associated with female sexual function complaints. In addition, the medications commonly used to treat depression can significantly affect the female sexual response. The most frequently used medications for uncomplicated depression are the selective serotonin re-uptake inhibitors (SSRIs).

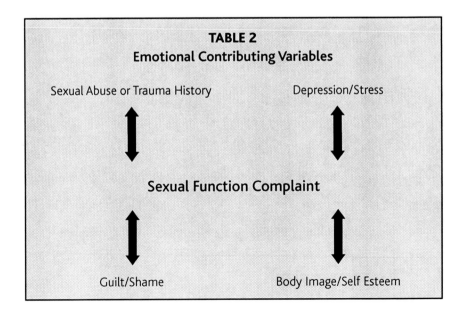

**TABLE 2**
**Emotional Contributing Variables**

Sexual Abuse or Trauma History          Depression/Stress

**Sexual Function Complaint**

Guilt/Shame          Body Image/Self Esteem

Women receiving these medications often complain of decreased desire, decreased arousal, decreased genital sensation, and difficulty achieving orgasm.

## IV. Assessment

All women are at risk for sexual dysfunction. If a physician is perceived as open to hearing about these complaints, it is more likely that the patient will bring them up during an exam. It is crucial, therefore, that the clinician provide appropriate cues that he or she is open to a discussion of sexual concerns. This can be achieved in many ways; the doctor may give the patient a sexual function questionnaire along with their paper work, or just include a question like, "Do you have any questions or concerns about your sexual response or interest," in the history. It is also helpful to place flyers or booklets about sexual function in the waiting and exam rooms to let your patients know you are receptive to hearing their concerns. In assessing a specific sexual concern raised by the patient, a more detailed history is appropriate (**See Table 3**).

A problem-solving approach to the patient's sexual complaint is recommended to clarify whether the complaint relates to desire, arousal, orgasm, or discomfort. Specific questions can assess the presence of a dysphoric disorder and a history of medication ingestion. Intrapsychic factors

---

**TABLE 3**
**Brief Clarification of a Sexual Concern in a Medical Practice**

- Clarify the problem (e.g. details, history, past attempts at treatment, etc.)
- Determine onset (gradual, acute, lifelong)
- Determine context for the complaints (generalized or situational)
- List all sexual symptoms
- Go over patient's typical sexual response cycle
- Consider partner reaction to the sexual dysfunction (level of conflict, stress, etc.)
- Couple motivation for treatment
- Medical, psychiatric and surgical history

of particular importance include stress, fatigue, depression, and substance abuse. Questions about the patient's early sex life may reveal a life-long inhibited sexual desire, sexual avoidance, or a history of childhood sexual trauma or abuse. If trauma or abuse history is discovered, it is crucial to send the patient for further support and evaluation by a trained therapist.

Relationship factors should be assessed for their relevant impact on the presenting complaint. Issues of grief, power, intimacy, and communication each require assessment to clarify whether the sexual concern is recent or a product of more serious longstanding conflicts. The physician's comfort in exploring these issues is most important. A relaxed physician in a comfortable atmosphere will encourage full disclosure by the patient. Staccato questions that run through a list of issues will likely yield little information and much frustration. If time is a factor, the assessment can be done over several visits. These complaints are rarely an emergency and may be better dealt with over more than one visit, as long as the second visit is not long after the first.

## Medical Tests

To understand what role physiologic factors may play in a woman's ability to respond sexually, the physician should conduct a full medical and surgical history with the patient. In addition, a hormonal profile is crucial in assessing the role of hormones in a woman's sexual function. Birth control pills, chronic stress, depression, and childbirth can all contribute to response, as well as, desire problems. A complete hormonal profile should include follicle-stimulating hormone, lutenizing hormone, testosterone (free and total), and estradiol levels. Medications or medical conditions that adversely affect libido or sexual function should be noted (see Table 4 for a complete list of medications that may affect sexual function).

The internal and external genitalia should also be thoroughly examined for signs of phlogosis, which can lead to vulvar pain in younger women as well as vaginal atrophy, pain, and arousal disorders in older menopausal women. The muscular tone and strength of the pelvic floor as well as the bulbocavernosus reflex should also be determined. Assessment of the genital and perineal sensation should be performed. If abnormalities are noted, further neurologic evaluation may be warranted.

It is important in some circumstances to also assess physiologic changes that occur during the sexual response. Measurements of genital vibratory

| TABLE 4 | |
| --- | --- |
| **Common Classes of Medications with Sexual Side Effect** | |
| Antihypersensitive Agents | Alpha–1 and –2 blockers (clonidine, reserpine, prazosin) |
| | Beta-blockers (metoprolol, propranolol) |
| | Calcium-channel blockers (diltiazem, nifedipine) |
| Chemotherapeutic Agents | Alkylating agents (busulfan, chlorambucil, cyclophosphamide) |
| CNS Agents | Anticholinergics (diphenhydramine) |
| | Anticonvulsants (carbamazepine, phenobarbital, phenytoin) |
| | Antidepressants (MAOIs, TCAs, SSRIs) |
| | Antipsychotics (phenothiazines, butyrophenones) |
| | Narcotics (oxycodone) |
| | Sedatives/anxiolyics (benzodiazephines) |
| Agents that Effect Hormones | Anti-androgens (cimetidine, spironolactone) |
| | Anti-estrogens (tamoxifen, raloxifene) |
| | Oral contraceptives |

perception thresholds and genital hemodynamics can be recorded post-sexual stimulation in the clinical setting. Blood flow assessment, especially clitoral, labial, urethral, vaginal and uterine arteries, is recorded and an assessment of blood velocity and venous pooling can be made. In many patients, observations show that despite complaints of sexual dysfunction, sexual stimulation does, in fact, result in significant increases in genital blood flow (Berman 1999). Currently, normative data is being gathered to determine normal physiologic responses.

## V. Therapies

### A. Biological and Physical Interventions

#### 1. Hormone therapy

##### a. Estrogen therapy

Estrogen therapy has many advantages. Recently, however, The National Institute of Health halted a longitudinal hormone

replacement study on the basis that there was increased risk for heart disease and breast cancer and ovarian cancer (Rossouw et al. 2002; Grady et al. 2002; Hulley et al. 2002; Lacey et al. 2002). As a result, patients are now closely involved in the decision making process and it is the responsibility of the physician to thoroughly discuss the options and risks with patients and help them make informed decisions.

In many instances, a safer and more effective medication could be prescribed in lieu of HRT, such as raloxifene or a bisphosphonate for bone demineralization, statins for lipid disorders, and aspirin for coronary heart disease and stroke prevention. It is important to educate patients as to the level of increased risks.

The bottom line is that the doctor must help each woman weigh the risks and benefits of HRT. Estrogen may relieve hot flashes, improve clitoral sensitivity, increase libido, and decrease pain and burning during intercourse. Local or topical estrogen application relieves symptoms of vaginal dryness, burning, and urinary frequency/urgency. In peri-menopausal, menopausal, or oophorectomized women, complaints of vaginal irritation, pain, or dryness may be relieved locally with low dose topical estrogen cream, vaginal estradiol rings or vaginal estradiol pellets, which may help to minimize the risks of estrogen.

b. Testosterone

The only FDA approved testosterone replacement available to women is methyltestosterone, indicated for menopausal women, used in combination with estrogen (Estratest), for symptoms of inhibited desire, dyspareunia, or lack of vaginal lubrication, as well as for its vaso-protective effects. A testosterone patch is presently being tested, and early trials indicate the patch may improve sexual activity as well as help create overall sense of well being (Shifren et al. 2000). According to the Princeton Consensus Panel on Female Androgen Insufficiency, if a woman exhibits symptoms of low testosterone (e.g. low libido, decreased energy and wellbeing), it is important to first determine an alternative explanation for these symptoms. This means ruling out major depression, chronic fatigue symptoms, as well as the range of other emotional and relationship conflicts that may impact on a patient's desire and happiness. The next step is to determine if the patient is in an adequate estrogen state, and if not, consider the pros and cons of replacement (Bachmann et al. 2002).

The physician should measure the patient's testosterone levels, which should include at least 2–3 measures of total and free testosterone. Normal value ranges are for total testosterone, 30–120 ng/dL, and for free testosterone, 3.0–8.5 pg/mL for pre-menopausal women and 3.0–6.7 pg/mL for post-menopausal women. If the patient has a treatable cause for the androgen deficiency (e.g. oral estrogens or contraceptive use) treat the specific causes by changing medications. If not, consider a trial of androgen replacement therapy.

There are conflicting reports regarding the best way to use testosterone, in particular in pre-menopausal women. Any pre-menopausal woman treated with testosterone must be on some form of reliable birth control and understand the risks. Topical vaginal testosterone is often used in pre-menopausal women as a first step in the treatment of sexual dysfunction and vaginal lichen planus. Topical testosterone (methyltestosterone or testosterone proprionate) preparations can be compounded in 1–2% formulations and should be applied up to three times per week. The suggested dose of oral testosterone (pill or sublingual spray or lozenge) for pre- and post-menopausal women ranges from .25–1.25 mg/day. The dose can be adjusted according to symptoms, free testosterone levels, cholesterol levels, triglyceride levels, HDL levels, and liver function test. The potential side effects of testosterone include weight gain, clitoral enlargement, increased facial hair, and hypercholesterolemia. Testosterone can also be converted into Estrogen, so physicians should take this risk into account when counseling their patients. Increased clitoral sensitivity, decreased vaginal dryness, and increased libido have been reported with the use of a 2% testosterone cream.

## 2. Pharmacological therapy

Aside from hormone replacement therapy, all medications listed below, while used in the treatment of male erectile dysfunction, are still in the experimental phases for use in women. Currently, we have limited information regarding the exact neurotransmitters that modulate vaginal and clitoral smooth muscle tone. Nitric oxide (NO) and Phosphodiesterase Type 5 (PDE5), the enzyme responsible for both the degradation of cGMP and NO production, have been identified in clitoral and vaginal smooth muscle (Liese et al. 1987). In addition, organ bath studies of rabbit clitoral, cavernosal muscle strips demonstrate enhanced relaxation in response to the nitric oxide donors, sodium nitroprusside, L-Arginine, and sildenafil.

a. Sildenafil

Functioning as a selective type 5 (cGMP specific) phosphodiesterase inhibitor, this medication decreases the catabolism of cGMP, the second messenger in nitric oxide mediated relaxation of clitoral and vaginal smooth muscle. Sildenafil may prove useful alone or possibly in combination with other vasoactive substances for treatment of female sexual arousal disorder. Two recent placebo controlled studies demonstrated that Sildenafil is successful in treating female sexual arousal disorder in hormonally replete women without psychosexual causal factors (Caruso 2001; Berman et al. 2003). However, Phase II clinical trials were halted. The company conducting the research reported that they were not finding a difference in effectiveness between Sildenafil and placebo, but this was most likely due to difficulties recruiting appropriate candidates. It proved difficult to identify women who did not have emotional or relationship causal factors influencing their sexual functioning, much less women who were hormonally replete with both estrogen and testosterone. Other studies have found that Sildenafil helps to alleviate arousal problems associated with aging, menopause, and arousal problems experienced secondary to selective serotonin re-uptake inhibitors (SSRI) use (Kim et al. 2000).

Sildenafil and other vasodilators will likely have their place as part of a multi-disciplinary treatment plan with a certain kind of candidate. These are most likely women who are hormonally replete and were satisfied with their sexual response at one point in time and now, for medical reasons (hysterectomy, menopause, pelvic injury, etc.) are no longer able to respond as they once could.

b. L-Arginine

This amino acid functions as a precursor to the formation of nitric oxide, which mediates the relaxation of vascular and non-vascular smooth muscle. L-Arginine has not yet been used in clinical trials in women. However, preliminary studies in men appear promising. A combination of L-Arginine and yohimbine (an alpha 2 blocker) is currently under investigation in women.

c. Yohimbine

Yohimbine is an alkaloid agent that blocks presynaptic alpha–2 adrenoreceptors. This medication affects the peripheral autonomic nervous system, resulting in a relative decrease in adrenergic activity and an increase in parasympathetic tone. There have been mixed reports of its efficacy for inducing penile erections in men, and formal clinical studies have not been performed in women to date, nor have potential side effects been effectively determined.

d. Prostaglandin $E_1$ (MUSE)

An intra-urethral application, absorbed via mucosa (MUSE), is now available for male patients. A similar application of Prostaglandin $E_1$ delivered intra-vaginally is currently under investigation for use in women. Clinical studies are necessary to determine the efficacy of this medication in the treatment of female sexual dysfunction.

e. Phentolamine

Currently available in an oral preparation, this drug functions as a non-specific alpha-adrenergic blocker, and causes vascular smooth muscle relaxation. This drug has been studied in male patients for the treatment of erectile dysfunction. A pilot study in menopausal women with sexual dysfunction demonstrated enhanced vaginal blood flow and subjective arousal with the medication (Rosen et al. 1999).

f. Apomorphine

This short acting dopamine agonist facilitates erectile responses in both normal males and males with psychogenic erectile dysfunction or organic impotence. Data suggests that dopamine is involved in the mediation of sexual desire and arousal. The physiologic effects of this drug are currently being tested in women with sexual dysfunction.

g. Nitroglycerin

Nitroglycerin (glyceryl trinitrate) has been used for over a century to relieve anginal symptoms associated with coronary artery disease. It has been administered to humans via oral, sublingual, intravenous, and transdermal routes. Nitroglycerin has been found to relax most smooth muscle, including bronchial, gastrointestinal tract, urethral, and uterine muscle. It also produces dilation of both arterial and venous vascular beds. Metabolism of nitroglycerin leads to the formation of the reactive free radical nitric oxide. Recent evidence suggests that application of nitroglycerin to painful areas, including the genitals, may provide analgesia to the affected areas (Walsh et al. 2002; Berrazueta et al. 1996). More work needs to be done in this area, but many experts are finding this an effective treatment for helping women manage vulvar pain, especially when in combination with topical estrogen and testosterone creams, and gynecological physical therapy.

### 3. Medical devices

a. Eros Therapy

Eros Therapy is the first FDA-approved treatment on the market for arousal and orgasmic disorders in women. It is a small, handheld medical device with a soft cup, which is placed over the clitoris. When activated, a gentle vacuum is created thereby increasing blood flow to the clitoris and surrounding tissue. Initial clinical trials showed improvement in pre- and post-menopausal women with female sexual arousal disorder or female orgasmic disorder (Billups et al. 2001; Berman et al. 2001).

b. InterStim Therapy

InterStim Therapy, a technique of implanting a neurostimulator with leads to the sacral nerve roots of S2 through S4, was originally designed to treat recalcitrant cases of urinary incontinence and other chronic bladder dysfunctions. Some women have reported anecdotally that they have experienced an increased sexual response following the placement of the InterStim. Further study of the use of InterStim for sexual enhancement is warranted.

### 4. Gynecological physical therapy

Chronic sexual pain disorders can effectively be treated with the use of gynecological physical therapy. With the use of manual therapies (internal or external), electrical therapy, exercise, and pelvic floor retraining, normal muscle balance, as well as bowel and bladder function can be restored, all of which results in improved sexual function. Physical therapy can also be helpful with issues of vaginal organ prolapse, rectal and fecal incontinence, and rectal pain.

### B. Psychosocial Interventions: the Role of Psychotherapy

As was mentioned above, more often than not, there are psychological and relationship factors contributing to a sexual problem. Even if the primary etiologic domain is physical, there are emotional and relationship outgrowths to the problem which cannot be ignored. Similarly, not all women are candidates for medical intervention and are better suited to other psychological or couples therapies (Billups et al. 2001; Berman et al. 2001). Usually the best treatment is a combination of medical interventions and psychotherapy. It should be noted here, that beginning psychotherapy without evaluating the potential medical causes for female sexual dysfunction is not recommended. Extensive psychotherapy with a woman with undiagnosed medical issues can be a very frustrating experience for both the patient and caregiver.

The ideal way to determine candidates for medical intervention in a clinical setting is to collaborate with a trained sex therapist. If the medical practitioner has access to a therapist on site, evaluation and diagnosis is optimized. Unfortunately, not all physicians have access to or facilities for incorporating a sex therapist into their practice. In this case, it is crucial for the physician to carry out an extensive assessment of the sexual complaints and the context in which they are experienced. This process not only entails a good global history, it also includes clarification of the sexual concern in a way that allows psychosexual red flags to be identified so that an appropriate therapy referral can be made (**see Table 5**).

**TABLE 5**
**Psychosexual Red Flags for Further Assessment***

- The symptoms are life long, not acquired
- The symptoms are situational (e.g. don't exist when stress removed or when with another partner)
- The patient has a history of sexual abuse or trauma
- The patient has a psychiatric history
- The patient has a history of or is presently experiencing depression and/or anxiety or stress
- The couple experiences relationship conflicts (e.g. lack of intimacy, conflict, etc.)
- The partner has a sexual dysfunction

*None of these factors guarantee the problem is psychosexually based, but simply point to a need for further clarification by a trained sex therapist

The key to making a therapy referral is in helping the patient understand where psychotherapy fits into the treatment equation. It may need to be clarified that, while you do not think her problems are "all in her head," she would benefit from psychotherapy as well as medical treatment. If the physician refers to and supports the role of the psychotherapy and helps the patient understand how psychotherapy will be incorporated in to her treatment plan, she will feel validated and encouraged, knowing that her symptoms will be addressed rather than minimized.

## VI. Conclusion

The ideal approach to female sexual health is a collaborative effort between physicians and therapists and should include a complete medical and psychosocial evaluation. Although there are significant anatomic and embryological parallels between men and women, the multifaceted nature of female sexual dysfunction is clearly distinct from that of the male. Frequently, the emotional and relationship well being a woman experiences contributes more to her sexual enjoyment than does her physiological response. These issues need to be addressed in conjunction with medical therapy in order for treatment to be effective. The presence of organic disease is often accompanied by psychosocial, emotional and/or relational factors that contribute to female sexual dysfunction. For this reason, a comprehensive approach, addressing both psychological as well as physiologic factors, is instrumental to the evaluation of female patients with sexual complaints

# *References*

Bachmann G, Bancroft J, Braunstein G, et al: Female androgen insufficiency: the princeton consensus statement on definition, classification, and assessment. Fertil Steril 77(4):660–65, 2002

Basson R, Berman J, Burnett A, et al: Report of the international consensus development conference on female sexual dysfunction: definitions and classifications. J Urol 163:889–93, 2000

Bengtson J: The Vagina. In KJ Ryan, RS Berkowitz, RL Barbieri, ed: Kitner's Gynecology. Mosbey, St Louis, 1995

Berman J, Berman: For Women Only. Henry Holt and Company, New York, 2001

Berman JR, Berman LA, Goldstein I: Female sexual dysfunction. Med Aspects Hum Sex 1(5):15, 1998

Berman JR, Berman LA, Toler SM et al: Safety and efficacy of sildenafil citrate for the treatment of female sexual arousal disorder: a double-blind, placebo controlled study. J Urol 170:2333–38, 2003

Berman L, Berman J, Chabra S, et al: Seeking help for sexual function complaints: what gynecologists need to know about the female patient's experience. Fertil Steril 79(3):572–76, 2003

Berman LA, Berman JR, Bruck D, et al: Pharmacology or psychotherapy?: effective treatment for fsd related to unresolved childhood sexual abuse. J Sex Marital Ther 27:421–25, 2001

Berman, JR, Berman LA, Goldstein I: Female sexual dysfunction: incidence, pathophysiology, evaluation and treatment options. Urology 54(3): 385–89, 1999

Berrazueta, JR, Losada, A, Poveda, J, et al: Successful treatment of shoulder pain syndrome due to supraspinatus tendonitis with transdermal nitroglycerin: a double blind study. Pain 66(1):63–67, 1996

Billups KL, Berman L, Berman J, et al: A new non-pharmacological vacuum therapy for female sexual dysfunction. J Sex Marital Ther 27(5):435–41, 2001

Caruso, S: Premenopausal women affected by sexual arousal disorder treated with sildenafil: a double-blind, cross-over, placebo-controlled study. Br J Obstet Gynaecol (108):623–28, 2001

Goldstein I, Berman J: Vasculogenic female sexual dysfunction: vaginal engorgement and clitoral erectile insufficiency syndromes. Int J Impot Res 10(2):S84–90, 1998

Goldstein I, Park, Tarcan T, et al: Histomorphometric analysis of age-related structural changes in human clitoral cavernosal tissue. J Urol 161:940–44, 1999

Grady D, Herrington D, Blumenthal R, et al: Cardiovascular disease outcomes during 6.8 years of hormone therapy: Heart and Estrogen/Progestin Replacement Study Follow-up (HERS II). JAMA 288:49–57, 2002

Graziottin A: Libido. In John Studd (ed): Yearbook of the Royal College of Obstetricians and Gynecologists, RCOG Press-Parthenon Publishing Group 235–243, 1996

Haefner H, Collins ME, Davis GD et al: Vulvar Pain Guideline. Journal of Lower Genital Tract Disease. In press, 2004

Harlow BL, Stewart EG: A population-based assessment of chronic unexplained vulvar pain: have we underestimated the prevalence of vulvodynia? J Am Med Womens Assoc 58:82–88, 2003

Hsueh WA: Sexual dysfunction with aging and systemic hypertension. American J Cardiol 61:18H–23H, 1998

Hulley S, Furberg C, Barrett-Connor E, et al: Noncardiovascular disease outcomes during 6.8 years of hormone therapy: Heart and Estrogen/ Progestin Replacement Study Follow-up (HERS II). JAMA 288:58–66, 2002

Kaplan HS: The New Sex Therapy. Bailliere Tindall, London, 1974

Kim NN, McAuley I, Min K, et al. Sildenafil augments pelvic nerve-mediated female genital sexual arousal in the anesthetized rabbit. Int J Impot Res 12, Suppl 3:S32-S39, 2001

Lacey JV, Mink PJ, Lubin JH, et al: Menopausal hormone replacement therapy and risk of ovarian cancer. JAMA 288:334–41, 2002

Lamont JA: Anorgasmia. Contemporary Obstetric Gynecology November:30, 1994

Lamont JA: Dyspareunia and vaginismus. In Droegemueller W, Sciarra JJ (eds): Gynecology and Obstetrics. Philadelphia, JB Lippincott, 1990

Lamont JA: Female dyspareunia. Am J Obstet Gynecol 136(3):282–85

Laumann E, Paik A, Rosen R: Sexual dysfunction in the United States prevalence and predictors. JAMA 281:537–44, 1999

Liese B, Nease D: Perceptions and treatment of sexual problems. Fam Med 11:468–70, 1987

Masters EH, Johnson VE: Human Sexual Response. Philadelphia: Lippincott Williams and Wilkins, 1966

McKay, M. Subsets of vulvodynia. J Repro Med 33(8):695–98, 1988

Metz ME, Seifert MH: Differences in men's and women's sexual health needs and expectations of physicians. Can J Hum Sex 2:53, 1993

Rosen RC, Phillips NA, Gendrano N: Oral phentolamine and female sexual arousal disorder: a pilot study. J Sex Marital Ther 25:137–44, 1999

Rossouw JE, Anderson GL, Prentice Rl, et al: Risks and benefits of estrogen plus progestin in healthy postmenopausal women: principal results from the women's health initiative randomized controlled trial. JAMA 288(3):321–33, 2002

Shifren JL, Braunstein GD, Simon JA, et al: Transdermal testosterone treatment in women with impaired sexual function after oopherectomy. N Engl J Med 343(10):682–88, 2000

Sipski ML, Alexander CJ, Rosen RC: Orgasm in women with spinal cord injuries: a laboratory-based assessment. Arch Phys Med Rehabil 75:1097–1102, 1995

Walsh KE, Berman JR, Berman LA, et al: Safety and efficacy of topical nitroglycerin for treatment of vulvar pain in women with vulvodynia: a pilot study. J Gend Specif Med 5:21–27, 2002

# 1

# Summary of Sex Surveys Findings

NATALYA BUSSEL, M.D.

## I. Introduction to Sex Surveys

In the United States, the Kinsey Report, one of the largest surveys was published in 1947. Alfred Kinsey, an evolutionary biologist and a professor of zoology from Indiana University, began studying human sexuality in 1938, when he was asked to teach the sexuality section of a course on marriage. Realizing the information on the topic was scarce; he initiated a survey by interviewing close to 18,000 subjects. Unfortunately, he was using samples of convenience including his own students, other college students, a group of homosexuals, mental hospital patients, etc. Samples of convenience, obviously, do not represent the behavior of the entire population (Bradburn and Sudman 1988). Kinsey published two books "Sexual Behavior in the Human Male" and "Sexual Behavior in the Human

Female." Kinsey statistics reported that 50% admitted that they committed adultery before turning 40 years old, 86% of men said they had engaged in premarital sex, half of the women who married after WWI were not virgins on their wedding day, 37% of men had at least one episode of sex with a male and 10% of men had had sex exclusively with other men for at least 3 years. Kinsey's findings shocked a conservative nation but his goal was to accumulate "scientific fact divorced from questions of moral value and social custom."

In the early 60s, gynecologist William Masters and his research associate Virginia Johnson initiated studying sexual behavior by bringing sex to the lab using a medical model. After witnessing a significant number of sexual encounters and using measurement methods, Masters and Johnson recorded their findings in books: "Human Sexual Response" (1966) and "Human Sexual Inadequacy" (1970) and "Homosexuality in Perspective" (1979).

The Playboy report is an example of many popular non-scientific attempts to gather data about sexual behavior in the post-Kinsey report era. Shere Hite sent out surveys to women whose names were obtained from women's organizations and subscribers to women's magazines. She distributed 100,000 questionnaires and got 3,000 back with a 3% response rate (Hite 1976). Similarly, 2% of the readers returned a survey sent to 4,700,000 Redbook readers. The small percentage of responders cast some doubts about the representative abilities of the findings.

The Janus Report, by Samuel S. Janus and Cynthia L. Janus was distributed to 4,550 subjects with 2,795 returned and were "satisfactorily completed" (Janus and Janus 1993). They reported that over 70% of Americans ages 65 and older have sex once a week. But the General Social Survey found that just 7% of older Americans have sex that often.

The AIDS crisis led to the creation of scientifically valid surveys worldwide. (French National Survey of Sexual Behavior–1998; Survey on Sexual Behavior in Japan, 1999, National Survey of Sexual Attitudes and Lifestyle in Britain, 1998, National Survey of sexual Attitudes of Czech Republic, 1997, Women's health Study–USA, 1997, New Zealand Partner Relations Survey, 1993, Alan Guttmacher Institute Surveys, Multiple National Surveys of Family Growth, NSFG, Multiple General Social Surveys, USA, National Surveys of Family and Households, USA, Several National Danish Surveys, Surveys on Adolescent Sexual Behavior and many others).

In 1990, The National Health and Social Life Survey (NHSLS) often called the Chicago Study or Chicago Survey, interviewed randomly selected 3,432 subjects with an age range of 18 to 59, and administered a face-to-face ninety-minute survey. The results of the study were published in Sex in America: a Definitive Survey (Michael et al. 1994), and The Social Organization of Sexuality (Laumann et al. 1994). NHSLS researchers were able to report on how often do people have sexual fantasies, how frequent they masturbate or have sex, etc. More findings from this survey are highlighted in this chapter. The survey also revealed that about 43% of women and 31% of men are suffering from sexual dysfunction. The specific findings of the prevalence of sexual disorders are listed for each specific disorder in the Epidemiology section.

## II. Sex Surveys Findings

### A. Frequency of Sexual Fantasies

NHSLS survey showed that 54% of men and 19% of women think about sex every day or several times daily. 43% of men and 67% of women think about it a few times a month or a week. 4% of men and 1% of women think about it less than once a month or never. 84% of married couples fantasize during intercourse. Most common fantasy content is having sex with loved one followed by having sex with a stranger, having sex with more than one person at same time, doing sexual things one would never do in reality, being forced to have sex forcing someone to have sex, having sex with someone of same gender (if hetero), and having sex with opposite sex (if lesbian/gay).

### B. Masturbation

According to NHSLS data, the frequency of masturbation is 40% in women and 60% of men in the past year. For married couples, the rates increase in men to 85% and to 45% in women in the past year.

### C. Frequency of Sexual Intercourse

The data from NHSLS showed that about a third have sex with partner at least twice a week, a third have sex a few times a month, and the rest have it a few times a year or have no sexual partners at all. The youngest and the oldest people in the NHSLS survey had the least sex with a partner. People in their twenties had the most. For both men and women, married and cohabiting couples are having the most sex. The frequency did not change with race, religion, or education. Data from surveys say that 40% of married people and half of people who are living together have sex 2 or more times a week. Less than 25% of single or dating men and women have sex 2 or more times a week. 25% of single people not living together reported to have sex just a few times a year and only about one in ten married people has sex at that frequency.

### D. Homosexuality

In 1973, homosexuality was eliminated as a diagnosed category by the American Psychiatric Association, and in 1980, it was removed from DSM. Judd Marmor, MD, was a key figure in "depathologizing" homosexuality as a character defect and its removal from APA Diagnostic and Statistical Manual. His two books about homosexuality "Sexual Inversion: The Multiple Roots of Homosexuality" (1965) and "Homosexual Behavior: A Modern Reappraisal (1980) brought a new perspective in this issue. However, from 1972 until 1991, polls conducted in the United States showed that over 70% of Americans believed that homosexuality was always morally wrong, which affected both what people say about their sexual behavior and what they actually do.

According to the Chicago Survey, 9 percent of men in the US twelve largest cities identify themselves as gay. But just 3 or 4% of the men living in the suburbs of these cities or other cities of the nation say they are gay and about 1% of men in rural areas identify themselves as gay. Lesbians tend to cluster in cities as well. The widely quoted figure, that 10% of Americans are homosexual, often attributed to Alfred Kinsey. However Kinsey emphasized that there is no single measure of homosexuality and that it is impossible to divide the world in two distinct classes—homosexuals and heterosexuals. He reported in 1948 that 37% of the white men he interviewed had had at least one sexual experience with another man in their lifetime. He then reported that from these same men 10% had only homosexual experiences for any three-year period between age 16 and 55. Kinsey published that about 13% of women have had at least one homosexual experience.

A 1994 survey of the U.S. Bureau of the Census concluded that the male prevalence rate of homosexuality is 2 to 3 percent. Data reported by The Wall Street Journal and The New York Times in 1993 from research studies on homosexual behavior worldwide, demonstrate that in Canada, in a sample of 5,514 first-year students college students under the age of 25 were 1% bisexual and 1% homosexual. In Norway, in a sample of 6,155 adults ages 18–26, 3.5% of males and 3% of females reported past homosexual experience. In France, in a sample of 20,055 adults, lifetime homosexual experience was reported in 4.1% of men and 2.6% of women. In Denmark, in a sample of 3,178 adults ages 18–59, less the 1% of men were exclusively homosexual. In Britain, in a sample of 18,876 adults ages 16–59, 6.1% percent reported past homosexual experience. According to the latest General Social Survey in 2003, estimates of male to male sex in the past year was higher than in surveys conducted in 1996 (3.1–3.7% compared with 1.7–2.0% for earlier surveys.) Yet all the numbers are still lower then 10%.

NHSLS Researchers wrote that about 5.5% of the women found the thought of having sex with a female appealing or very appealing. About 4% of the women were sexually attracted to the same gender. Less than 2% of the women had sex with another woman in the past year, about 4% had sex with another woman after the age of 18, and a little more then 4% had sex with a woman at some time in their life. About 6% of the men were attracted to other men according to the same study. About 2% of the men had sex with a man in the past year, a little more then 5% had homosexual sex at least once since they turned 18. 40% of men had sex with another man before they are 18 years old. About 1.4% of women and about 2.8% of men identified themselves as homosexuals. In terms of numbers of gay and lesbians, the figures of the Chicago Survey were closer to the AIDS Surveys in the United States as well the Sexuality surveys in England and France.

The Chicago Survey, along with other studies in Europe, found that people who identify themselves as gays and lesbians tend to live in urban areas, and tend to be more highly educated. The data showed that twice as many college-educated men identify themselves as homosexual as opposed to men with high school education (3% and 1.5% respectively). Women with college educations are eight times more likely to identify themselves as lesbians as opposed to women with high-school education, 4% and 0.5% respectively (Michael et al. 1994; Laumann et al. 1994). At present, gay men and lesbians advocate new laws to protect them from discrimination in the workplace and housing, they want to be married, want to be given the same benefits as married couples and be allowed to adopt children.

Biological factors in homosexuality are still under study. Some studies have shown differences in size in the Sexually Dimorphic Nucleus (SDN) located in the Preoptic Area, and the Third Interstitial Nucleus of the Anterior Hypothalamus (INAH3), between heterosexuals and homosexuals. These studies are inconclusive and cannot yet be interpreted to support the biological etiology of homosexuality.

### E. Sexually Transmitted Diseases (STD)/AIDS

Medical scientists currently recognize at least 20 sexually transmitted diseases, including genital herpes, Chlamydia, HPV, Hepatitis B, Hepatitis C, and many others including, of course, AIDS. The Centers for Disease Control and Prevention asks doctors to report STD, but few private doctors do. Public clinics report them, but as cases, not as patients. That means that once a patient who got re-infected several times would be reported each time as a new case. Some STDs, even if they are dangerous, are not reportable. In addition, herpes infection tends to recur, and Chlamydia infections could be difficult to diagnose (needs definite laboratory tests). For all these reasons, the national statistics of STDs have been deficient. Overall researchers discovered that 18% of women and 16% of men have had an STD once in their life. It is important to know that women are more likely to have an STD than men. It reflects the medical finding that it is at least twice as easy for a man to infect a woman with virtually any STD including AIDS than it is for a woman to infect a man. Individuals with many partners, especially those who rarely use condoms, have as much as a ten-fold greater chance of being infected than do those with few or only one partner, i.e., risk growing with the number of partners (Michael et al. 1994).

AIDS high-risk groups are men who had sex with men, intravenous drug abusers; and their partners, and their children, hemophiliacs and others who had received contaminated blood products. With proper handling of the blood supply, the last group has decreased risk and pressing questions began to center on the other groups. AIDS is spread through sexual intercourse, and that it seems to spread more efficiently through anal intercourse that through vaginal intercourse. AIDS also is transmitted very efficiently when an infected intravenous drug user shares needles with people who are infected. It is important to know that the chances of male to female vaginal transmission after just one act of unprotected sex is 1/500, but women are less likely to transmit HIV to a man (1/2,000) as was estimated by scientists at the Centers for Disease Control and Prevention. The chance of the transmission decreasing also is if the infected person takes anti-retroviral medications. Since the end of WW II, intravenous drug use, largely heroin, was concentrated among poor people in the inner cities, men more likely than women. In many inner city neighborhoods such as New York, 50–75% of heroin users were infected with HIV (Michael et al. 1994). The World Health Organization estimates that more than 40,000,000 people worldwide are infected with HIV/AIDS.

The behavior of people has changed because of risks of AIDS and other STD. NHSLS researchers revealed that 27% of people who are at risk said that they had been tested. Those who tested tended to be younger, more educated, and living in largest cities; 30% of blacks, 26% of whites and 25% of Hispanics admitted to having been tested. Of those who currently were married, 23% had been tested, while 37% of cohabiting also had. Of those who were not cohabiting, 30% said they had been tested. There was no difference between the poor, the middle income, and the wealthy in the percentage, of who had been tested for HIV. It is important to notice that those who had been tested were with disproportionably many sex partners since the age of 18 and more partners within the past twelve months (Michael et al. 1994; Laumann et al. 1994).

According to NHSLS, 30% of people at risk admitted to change their risky sexual behavior. They tended to be younger and living in large cities. There was no pattern by education or income level, but 46% of blacks, 37% of Hispanics and 26% of whites said that they changed their behavior. Only 12% of the married respondents had changed their behavior, while 40% of cohabiting and 32% of non-cohabiting respondents had done so. Again, the stronger patterns were by number of partners, those who had zero or one partner since the age of 18, changed their behavior only in 10% of cases comparing to 76% of those with "five or more" partners over the past year (Michael et al. 1994; Laumann et al. 1994).

The Alan Guttmacher Institute reported an increase of condom use from 13% to 19% of all women and was higher among women younger than 20 years of age than among those aged 30 years or older. The condom use was most common among those never married who were not cohabiting. Women in early stage of relationship (six months or less) were using condoms much more likely than those in a long-standing relationship (5 years or more (odds ratio, 1.5). Younger and better educated women were more likely to be currently using condoms than were older or less educated women. The national survey in Switzerland revealed the majority of respondents using protection (condoms)—between 16–20 years of age, adolescents (girls: 63%, boys: 58%). In Great Britain, the National Survey of Sexual Attitudes and Lifestyles (NATSAL) reported greater changes in sexual behavior for women than men. Researchers reported an increase of risky sexual behavior compared to previous years, but greater condom use. 2.6% of both men and women reported homosexual partnership; and 4.3% of men reported paying for sex. The National Household Survey in Spain, 3% reported engaging in HIV sexual risk behavior, having more than one partner and failure to use condoms systematically (they were mostly male, age 20–59 and unmarried. A survey in Sweden revealed changes in attitudes regarding HIV, but modest changes in sexual behavior, however increase in condom use, particularly in younger respondents, that may facilitate the prevention of HIV in Sweden. There are still countries where analysis keeps revealing poor levels of awareness on STDs and HIV/AIDS. For example, a survey in Nairobi, Kenya revealed both, no changes in sexual behavior, 75.9% of not using any protective measures against STD or HIV, and low awareness about STD, HIV/AIDS. AIDS epidemic is changing. It is starting to concentrate more in poor neighborhoods and less among gay men. Many gay men have changed their risky behavior, decreased attending bathhouses (being popular previously) after realization of the consequences of frequent unprotected sex (Laumann et al. 1994). National Survey in Denmark reported that Danish gay men increased sexual safety, but risky sex still prevails among substantial minority.

At the same time AIDS is becoming endemic in poor neighborhoods, among drug users and their sexual partners, where behavior has changed little (Laumann et al. 1994). Although STDs are a risk for sexually active people in any age group, teens and adolescents are particularly vulnerable because they tend to have more partners and because they are inconsistent in using protection. One in four sexually active teens acquires an STD. In a study of African-American women college students, 65% had never, or rarely used condoms, although they knew about condom effectiveness. Studies in many cultures show that large proportions of young heterosexuals still engage in unprotected sex. For example, a Nigerian study of a large sample of adolescents showed that only 21 percent of girls and 36 percent of boys used condoms, although they knew about condom effectiveness in STD prevention. Among teens in developed countries, the main reason for not using protection seems to be that safer sex inconsistent with the romantic, spontaneous sex of scripted fantasies. The strongest factors determining both men's and women's condom use was their concern that it would destroy the romance and their fear of negative implications College students underestimate the risk of AIDS because they use inaccurate decision rules; they may judge their risk of AIDS based on their partners' appearance.

The campaigns toward the increase the levels of education, increasing people's motivation to reduce their own risk, and teaching them the specific skills and behaviors should be continued all over the world. Counseling and education on sexuality should be a continuing process and require interdisciplinary training for professional team working in health care, services with an emphasis on sexual behavior, prevention, attitude and reproductive rights.

## F. Sexuality and Culture

Human sexuality is highly controlled by cultural norms. The concept of sexual scripts has been introduced to the literature. They set the standards for interpersonal behavior, e.g., on a first date, and they are influenced by race and class as well as by gender. Ethnic groups showed significant differences in sexual behavior. For example, compared with American college students, Chinese students start dating at a later age, date less often, and are less likely to have sex with their dates. More details about sexuality and culture are provided in Sex in America: A Definitive Survey (Michael et al. 1994).

## III. Conclusion

Sexual behavior is a complex topic with many misconceptions that are constantly challenged by accurate and valid survey studies. A complex web of cultural, social, interpersonal, psychological, and biological factors surround the topic of sex.

## *References*

Bradburn NM, S. Sudman S: Polls and Surveys: Understanding What They Tell Us. San Francisco, CA, Jossey-Bass Publishers, 1988

Hite S: The Hite Report. New York, Dell, 1976

Janus SS and Janus CL: The Janus Report on Sexual Behavior. New York, NY, John Wiley and Sons, 1993

Laumann EO, Gagnon JH, Michael RT, and Michaels S: The Social Organization of Sexuality: Sexual Practices in the United States. Chicago, IL, University of Chicago Press, 1994

Masters and Johnson, Human Sexual Response. Boston, Little Brown, 1966

Masters WH: Homosexuality in Perspective. Baltimore, MD, Lippincott Williams & Wilkins, 1979

Masters WH: Human Sexual Inadequacy. Baltimore, MD, Lippincott Williams & Wilkins, 1970

Michael RT, Gagnon JH, Laumann EO, and Kolata G: Sex in America: a Definitive Survey. New York, NY, Little Brown, 1994

# 2

# Screening Tests for Sexual Disorders

WAGUIH WILLIAM ISHAK, M.D.

## I. Online Sexual Disorders Screening for Women (Sadock and IsHak 1996)

1. I think or fantasize about sex:

   ❑ Not at all    ❑ Some of the time    ❑ Frequently    ❑ Almost Always

2. I am able to become aroused:

   ❑ Not at all    ❑ Some of the time    ❑ Frequently    ❑ Almost Always

3. I have a difficulty remaining aroused during sex:

   ❑ Not at all    ❑ Some of the time    ❑ Frequently    ❑ Almost Always

4. I experience vaginal lubrication during sex:

   ❑ Not at all    ❑ Some of the time    ❑ Frequently    ❑ Almost Always

5.  I have a difficulty reaching orgasm:

    ❏ Not at all    ❏ Some of the time    ❏ Frequently    ❏ Almost Always

6.  I enjoy having sex with my partner (if you have one):

    ❏ Not at all    ❏ Some of the time    ❏ Frequently    ❏ Almost Always

7.  I engage in masturbation more than I feel is normal:

    ❏ Not at all    ❏ Some of the time    ❏ Frequently    ❏ Almost Always

8.  I worry about my sexual responsiveness:

    ❏ Not at all    ❏ Some of the time    ❏ Frequently    ❏ Almost Always

9.  I feel frightened about having sex:

    ❏ Not at all    ❏ Some of the time    ❏ Frequently    ❏ Almost Always

10. I experience pain during intercourse:

    ❏ Not at all    ❏ Some of the time    ❏ Frequently    ❏ Almost Always

**Disclaimer:**

SDS is a preliminary screening test for sexual symptoms that does not replace in any way a formal psychiatric or medical evaluation. It is designed to give a preliminary idea about the presence of sexual symptoms that indicate the need for an evaluation by a psychiatrist or a physician.

## II. Online Sexual Disorders Screening for Men (Sadock and IsHak 1996)

1. I think or fantasize about sex:

   ❏ Not at all    ❏ Some of the time    ❏ Frequently    ❏ Almost Always

2. I am able to get an erection:

   ❏ Not at all    ❏ Some of the time    ❏ Frequently    ❏ Almost Always

3. I maintain an erection as long as I want to:

   ❏ Not at all    ❏ Some of the time    ❏ Frequently    ❏ Almost Always

4. I ejaculate before I want to:

   ❏ Not at all    ❏ Some of the time    ❏ Frequently    ❏ Almost Always

5. I have difficulty reaching a climax:

   ❏ Not at all    ❏ Some of the time    ❏ Frequently    ❏ Almost Always

6. I enjoy having sex with my partner (if you have one):

   ❏ Not at all    ❏ Some of the time    ❏ Frequently    ❏ Almost Always

7. I engage in masturbation more than I feel is normal:

   ❏ Not at all    ❏ Some of the time    ❏ Frequently    ❏ Almost Always

8. I worry about my sexual performance:

   ❏ Not at all    ❏ Some of the time    ❏ Frequently    ❏ Almost Always

9. I feel frightened about having sex:

   ❏ Not at all    ❏ Some of the time    ❏ Frequently    ❏ Almost Always

10. I experience pain when I have an erection or ejaculate:

    ❏ Not at all    ❏ Some of the time    ❏ Frequently    ❏ Almost Always

**Disclaimer:**

SDS is a preliminary screening test for sexual symptoms that does not replace in any way a formal psychiatric or medical evaluation. It is designed to give a preliminary idea about the presence of sexual symptoms that indicate the need for an evaluation by a psychiatrist or physician.

# *References*

Sadock BJ and IsHak WW: Online Sexual Disorders Screening
        for Women, NYU Department of Psychiatry,
            http://www.med.nyu.edu/psych/screens/sdsf.html, 1996
Sadock BJ and IsHak WW: Online Sexual Disorders
        Screening for Men, NYU Department of Psychiatry,
            http://www.med.nyu.edu/psych/screens/sdsm.html, 1996

3

# The DSM-IV in a Nutshell: A Practical Approach to Psychiatric Diagnosis

Waguih William IsHak, M.D., Eugene Lee, M.D.,
Ravi Bhalavat, M.D., Monisha Vasa, M.D.

## I. Introduction:

The Diagnostic and Statistical Manual of Mental Disorders, Fourth Edition, Text Revision (DSM-IV-TR) is the most commonly used diagnostic reference in psychiatry (APS 2000). The diagnostic process can be complicated and requires contemplation of broad differentials to account for the multiple symptoms patients may exhibit. There have been active attempts at simplifying DSM-IV-TR. "The DSM-IV in a Nutshell" is a stepwise decision tree to assist in formulating the psychiatric diagnosis. It neatly summarizes the DSM-IV-TR on one page (Figure 1). This approach to diagnosis includes a 3-step process:

**Step 1** to rule out disorders first diagnosed in childhood, disorders due to general medical conditions, and substance-induced disorders,

**Step 2** to scan five sets of Axis I disorders (Psychotic, Mood, Anxiety, Somatoform, or Other) each of which is contains six diagnoses, and then

**Step 3** to identify which personality disorder (if any) out of three clusters with total of ten personality disorders.

**Figure 1: The DSM-IV In a Nutshell** by Waguih William IsHak, MD, FAPA, Eugene Lee, MD, Ravi Bhalavat, MD, and Monisha Vasa, MD

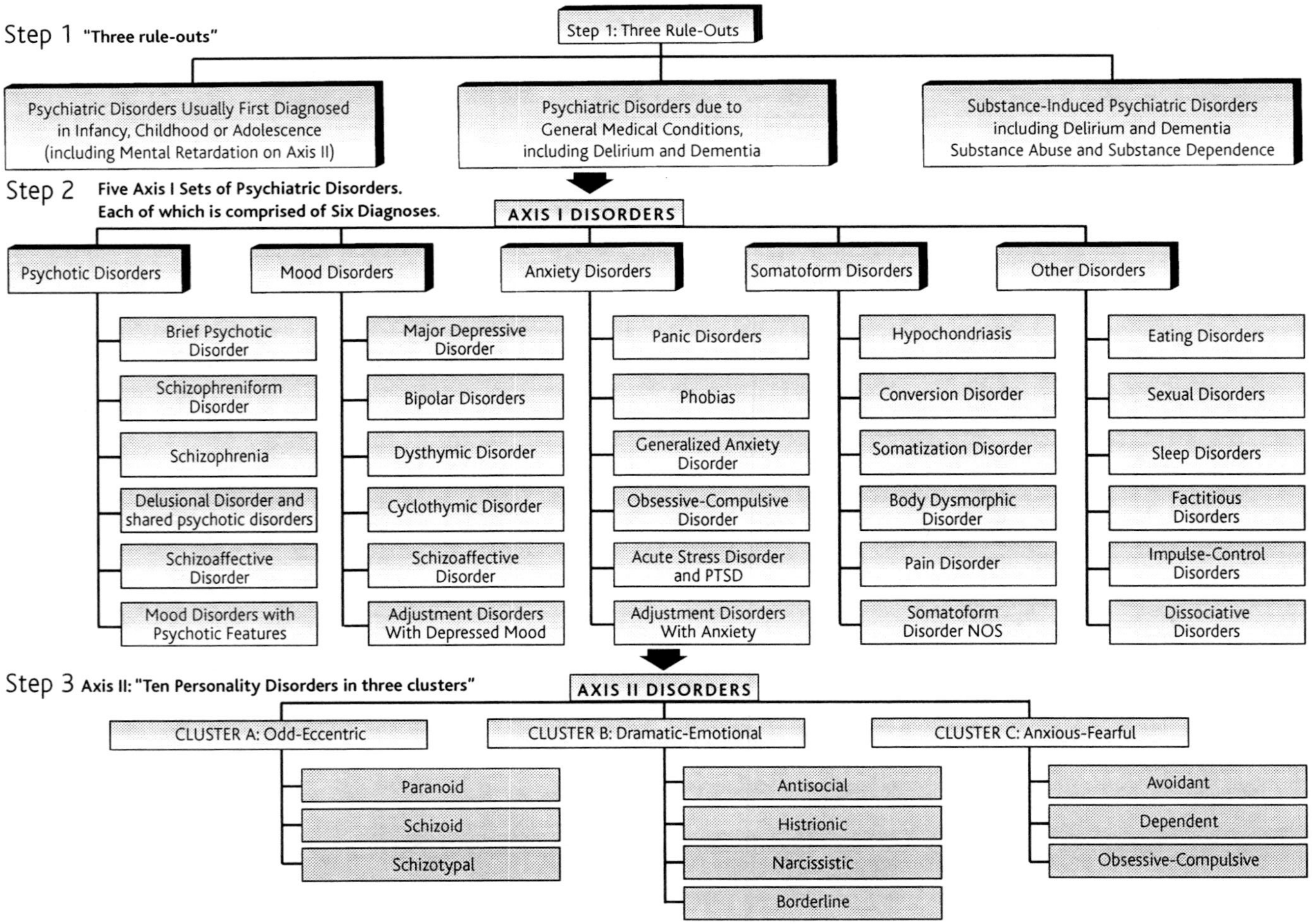

Step 1 "Three rule-outs"

Step 1: Three Rule-Outs

Psychiatric Disorders Usually First Diagnosed in Infancy, Childhood or Adolescence (including Mental Retardation on Axis II)

Psychiatric Disorders due to General Medical Conditions, including Delirium and Dementia

Substance-Induced Psychiatric Disorders including Delirium and Dementia Substance Abuse and Substance Dependence

Step 2    Five Axis I Sets of Psychiatric Disorders. Each of which is comprised of Six Diagnoses.

**AXIS I DISORDERS**

Psychotic Disorders
- Brief Psychotic Disorder
- Schizophreniform Disorder
- Schizophrenia
- Delusional Disorder and shared psychotic disorders
- Schizoaffective Disorder
- Mood Disorders with Psychotic Features

Mood Disorders
- Major Depressive Disorder
- Bipolar Disorders
- Dysthymic Disorder
- Cyclothymic Disorder
- Schizoaffective Disorder
- Adjustment Disorders With Depressed Mood

Anxiety Disorders
- Panic Disorders
- Phobias
- Generalized Anxiety Disorder
- Obsessive-Compulsive Disorder
- Acute Stress Disorder and PTSD
- Adjustment Disorders With Anxiety

Somatoform Disorders
- Hypochondriasis
- Conversion Disorder
- Somatization Disorder
- Body Dysmorphic Disorder
- Pain Disorder
- Somatoform Disorder NOS

Other Disorders
- Eating Disorders
- Sexual Disorders
- Sleep Disorders
- Factitious Disorders
- Impulse-Control Disorders
- Dissociative Disorders

Step 3  Axis II: "Ten Personality Disorders in three clusters"

**AXIS II DISORDERS**

CLUSTER A: Odd-Eccentric
- Paranoid
- Schizoid
- Schizotypal

CLUSTER B: Dramatic-Emotional
- Antisocial
- Histrionic
- Narcissistic
- Borderline

CLUSTER C: Anxious-Fearful
- Avoidant
- Dependent
- Obsessive-Compulsive

## II. Using "The DSM-IV in a Nutshell" Approach:

"The DSM-IV in a Nutshell" is a stepwise decision tree in order to reach a psychiatric diagnosis.

**Step One:** The three rule-outs:

- Disorders Usually First Diagnosed in Infancy, Childhood, or Adolescence,
- Disorders Due to General Medical Conditions
- Substance-Induced Psychiatric Disorders.

Any positive findings on these three rule-outs would require clinicians to examine the significance of their impact on the target psychiatric symptoms.

**Step Two:** Cover the five main sets of Axis I disorders. (A) Psychotic, (B) Mood, (C) Anxiety, (D) Somatoform, or (E) Other disorders. Each of these sets may be subdivided into six discrete diagnoses (labeled 1 through 6).

**(A) Psychotic Disorders**, as a group, are characterized by delusions, hallucinations, disorganized speech, disorganized behavior, or negative symptoms, as defined by Criterion A for Schizophrenia. The six Psychotic Disorders differ primarily in the duration of disturbance, or in the relationship of mood and psychotic symptoms. (1) Brief Psychotic Disorder lasts from one day to one month. (2) Schizophreniform Disorder lasts from one to six months. (3) Schizophrenia has continuous signs that persist for more than six months. (4) Delusional Disorder lasts at least one month and primarily involves nonbizarre delusions. (Consider Shared Psychotic Disorder if there is a close relationship with another person who already has an established delusion). The two remaining Psychotic Disorders differ by the relationship of psychosis to mood. In (5) Schizoaffective Disorder, psychosis persists for at least two weeks in the absence of prominent mood symptoms, whereas in (6) Mood Disorders with Psychotic Features, psychosis occurs only in the context of mood symptoms.

**(B) Mood Disorders** are characterized by the presence of mood symptoms: anhedonia or depressed mood for major depressive episodes, and irritable, expansive, or elevated mood for manic episodes. The six Mood Disorders also differ in duration, as well as severity, of disturbance. (1)

Major Depressive Disorder involves a Major Depressive Episode lasting at least two weeks in duration. (2) Bipolar Disorder involves a Manic Episode lasting at least one week in duration (or symptoms severe enough to require hospitalization). (3) Dysthymic Disorder involves low-grade depressive symptoms (more days than not) lasting two years (or one year in children and adolescents). (4) Cyclothymic Disorder involves cycling depressive and hypomanic symptoms lasting two years (or one year in children and adolescents). (5) Schizoaffective Disorder involves psychotic symptoms during and after mood episodes (remember also to consider Mood Disorders with Psychotic Features per psychotic differential above), and (6) the Adjustment Disorders are mood disturbances that occur within three months of an identifiable stressor(s). Note that the Adjustment Disorders may occur With Depressed Mood, With Anxiety, or With Mixed Anxiety and Depressed Mood.

**(C) Anxiety Disorders** are characterized by the presence of fears, worries, autonomic symptoms, and avoidance or compulsive behaviors. (1) Panic Disorder features Panic Attacks, and may occur with or without Agoraphobia. (2) Phobias involve fears, without apparent justification, of specific things, places, or situations. Phobias may be specific or social. (3) Generalized Anxiety Disorder involves excessive worries and fears (more days than not) for at least six months. (4) Obsessive-Compulsive Disorder involves recurrent, uncontrollable intrusive thoughts that are only relieved by compulsive behaviors. (5) Acute Stress Disorder follows a traumatic event and lasts two days to four weeks (if longer than one month, then consider Posttraumatic Stress Disorder). (6) And again, the Adjustment Disorders occur within three months of an identifiable stressor(s) and may occur With Depressed Mood, With Anxiety, or With Mixed Anxiety and Depressed Mood.

**(D) Somatoform Disorders** are characterized by preoccupation with the body (appearance or function) or having physical symptoms with no medical basis. (1) Hypochondriasis entails a fear of having serious disease based on the person's misinterpretation of bodily symptoms. (2) Conversion Disorder involves unintentional motor or sensory dysfunction suggesting a neurological or other general medical condition but associated with psychological factors. (3) Somatization Disorder involves symptoms grouped by system (at least 4 pain, 2 gastrointestinal, 1 sexual, and 1 pseudoneurological) as well as onset before age 30. (4) Body Dysmorphic Disorder is a preoccupation with an imagined defect in appearance. (5) Pain Disorder is physical pain where psychological factors are judged to play a significant role. (6) Somatoform Disorder NOS comprises patients who commonly do not fit criteria of the above five disorders (e.g., Somatization Disorder starting after age 30).

**(E) Other Disorders** are qualitatively different. The first three involve three bodily functions: (1) Eating Disorders, (2) Sexual (and Gender Identity) Disorders, and (3) Sleep Disorders. The last three have no common theme and would need to be memorized: (4) Factitious Disorders, (5) Impulse-Control Disorders, and (6) Dissociative Disorders.

<u>**Step Three**</u> is to identify any enduring patterns of inner experience and behavior that deviate markedly from the expectations of the individual's culture. If these patterns are inflexible and pervasive across a broad range of personal and social situations, and lead to clinically significant distress or impairment, then the patient may meet criteria for a Personality Disorder. Personality Disorders (PDs) are arranged in three Clusters: A, B, and C.

People living with **Cluster A PDs** often appear odd or eccentric. Paranoid PD involves distrust and suspiciousness that others' motives may be malevolent. Schizoid PD is a pattern of detachment from social relationships and a restricted range of emotional expression. Schizotypal PD implies acute discomfort in close relationships, cognitive or perceptual distortions, and eccentricities of behavior.

**Cluster B PDs** manifest in dramatic, emotional, or erratic behaviors. Antisocial personalities disregard and violate the rights of others. Borderline traits include impulsivity and instability in interpersonal relationships, self-image, and affect. Histrionic personality traits include excessive attention seeking and emotionality. People with Narcissistic PD can be grandiose, need admiration, and lack empathy.

**Cluster C PDs** often appear anxious or fearful. People with Avoidant PD feel inadequate, are socially inhibited, and hypersensitive to negative evaluation. Dependent personality traits include being are submissive and clingy, with an excessive need to be taken care of. Finally, Obsessive-Compulsive PD should not be confused with Obsessive-Compulsive Disorder: the former is a pattern of preoccupation with orderliness, perfectionism, and control, whereas the latter is an Axis I anxiety disorder involving intrusive thoughts and compulsive behaviors.

## III. Case Example:

A 31-year-old single, Caucasian female who was brought to the Emergency Department after a serious suicide attempt. Target symptoms included depressed mood, most of the day every day, for three weeks, with terminal insomnia, weight loss, guilt and low self-esteem, poor concentration, and continued suicidality. She had one prior depressive episode. She has no history of manic or psychotic symptoms. She experiences intense emotional reactions to people and events with severe concern about being abandoned and chronic feelings of emptiness. She cut her forearms to "feel something". She has no history of substance use and her urine drug screen was negative. Her medical history included migraine headaches.

An evaluating clinician could utilize the **"DSM-IV In a Nutshell"** to systematically assess her symptoms. Step 1 leads the clinician to evaluate substance-related disorders, which are ruled out based on history and labs. She did not have any symptoms that indicated a diagnosis first diagnosed in childhood. She did have migraines, but her symptoms were not a direct result of this medical condition. Step 2 leads the clinician to evaluate her symptoms via the "Mood" algorithm. She met criteria for a major depressive episode. Her lack of hypomanic or manic symptoms, as well as the duration and severity of her symptoms, ruled out the other mood disorders. She did not exhibit symptoms in the "Psychotic", "Anxiety", "Somatoform", or "Other" categories. Step 3 addressed her symptoms of mood reactivity, chronic emptiness, fear of abandonment, suicidality, and self-mutilatory behaviors. This would lead to a strong possibility of a cluster B Borderline Personality Disorder pending more information.

With this educational tool, the clinician could confidently and accurately diagnose "Major Depressive Disorder," and "Rule out Borderline Personality Disorder."

## IV. Conclusion

In summary, formulating and modifying the differential diagnosis is a critical step of every clinical encounter. Advantages of "The DSM-IV in a Nutshell" are that it is practical, convenient, and easy to remember. By no means does it seek to be complete; rather, it is a concise map of psychiatric diagnoses.

## *Refererence*

American Psychiatric Association (APA): Diagnostic and Statistical Manual of Mental Disorders, 4th ed. Text Revision, Washington, DC, American Psychiatric Publishing Inc., 2000.

# Index

## A

abreaction, 165, 167, 170
ACE-inhibitor, 53
acquired, 27, 32, 82, 116, 135, 136, 138, 142, 183, 194, 210
acquired type, 32, 116
acupuncture, xiv, 174, 175, 177, 178, 179, 180, 189
addiction, 97, 98, 99, 200
AIDS, 216, 219, 220, 221, 222, 223
alcohol, 28, 49, 53, 57, 58, 60, 61, 69, 78, 90, 106, 117, 200
alprostadil, 35, 79, 113, 120, 123
ambivalence, 154
amineptine, 55
Amyl Nitrate, 61
analgesics, 157
androgen, 47, 70
anemia, 23, 69, 90
anorgasmia, 46, 135, 138, 140, 141, 144, 195
anti-hypertensive, 49, 54
anticholinergic, 49, 55
antipsychotics, 49, 57, 90
anxiety, 49, 59, 70, 77, 82, 84, 90, 91, 92, 94, 95, 96, 98, 107, 129, 133, 138, 141, 144, 155, 156, 157, 159, 164, 165, 166, 183, 192, 200, 210

aphrodisiacs, 37, 182, 189
Apomorphine, 45, 112, 207
aromatherapy, 173, 174, 182
arousal, xi, 8, 9, 10, 15, 17, 27, 31, 35, 39, 50, 71, 103, 104, 116, 117, 123, 178, 194, 195
atherosclerosis, 23, 29, 52, 69, 70, 74, 77, 106, 118, 137, 197
autoimmune, 69
autonomic, 65, 75, 108, 130, 153, 154, 178, 179, 207
aversion, 88, 93, 94, 95, 96, 99, 100, 162, 194
Ayurvedic Medicine, 173, 185, 186

## B

Basson, Rosemary, 15
benzodiazepines, 49, 137
Berman, Jennifer and Laura, 4
biofeedback, 93, 166
biopsychosocial approach, 2, 87, 99
body image, 16, 70, 90, 138, 146, 154, 169, 200
Botulinium toxin, 165
bromocriptine, 71
Bupropion, 63, 92, 100
buspirone, 56

**235**

# C

cabergoline, 45, 71, 140, 144
Calcium Channel Blockers, (CCBs), 53
cancer, 48, 79, 80, 83, 120, 145, 151, 204, 212
cavernosometry, 30, 73, 110
Chinese herbs, 180
cholinergic, 45, 75, 108
chronic vulvar pain, 167, 195
Cialis *(see tadalafil)*
citalopram, 55, 130
climax, 131, 135, 227
clitoral, 71, 194
    blood flow, 23, 195, 197
    stimulation, 13, 135
clomipramine, 98, 131, 132
clozapine, 57
Cocaine, 50, 59, 65
CBT, 93, 96, 98, 170
cognitive behavioral therapy,
cognitive behavioral therapy (CBT), 93, 96, 98, 170
coital pain, 149
compulsive, 97, 98, 99, 100
condoms, 131
confidentiality, 25, 26, 192
congenital, 48, 69, 106
corpus cavernosum, 4, 33, 43, 52, 64, 66, 114
couple therapy, 24, 37, 166
cyclic-guanosine monophosphate, (cGMP), 107
cyproheptadine, 56
Cystocele, 83
cytokines, 76

# D

depression, 49, 54, 55, 70, 82, 90, 91, 92, 107, 118, 141, 200, 202, 204
desire, vii, xi, 8, 9, 10, 16, 17, 19, 27, 31, 50, 64, 68, 70, 87, 88, 89, 91, 97, 98, 99, 100, 178, 194

detumescence, 109
devices, 33, 35, 40, 78, 79, 81, 114, 115, 208
Diabetes, 23, 68, 74, 77, 78, 106, 129
Diabetes Mellitus, 23, 68, 106, 129
diuretics, 51, 52, 90
dopamine, 1, 45
Doppler imaging, 30
doxazosin, 34, 53
DSM-IV-TR, 8, 31, 67, 71, 81, 88, 104, 116, 125, 149, 150, 160, 167
Duplex Doppler, 119
Dyslipidemia, 75
Dyspareunia, 32, 68, 82, 90, 149, 150, 151, 153, 154, 159, 168, 169, 170, 171, 196, 212

# E

ejaculation, 13, 32, 61, 81, 125, 126, 127, 145, 148, 186
ejaculatory latency, 126, 128, 131
endocrine, 45, 63, 81, 109, 179, 194
endometriosis, 69, 72, 153, 156, 197
endorphins, 12
endothelial dysfunction, 74, 75
Engel, George, 21
ephedrine, 56, 57, 60, 65
erection, 11, 107
Eros Clitoral Therapy Device, 120, 139
erotic, 38, 65, 108, 139, 165, 182, 183, 184
estrogen, 48, 70, 92, 120, 152, 199, 203, 204, 205, 212
ethanol, 57
excitement, 8, 10, 17

# F

fantasies, 11, 70, 88, 89, 194, 217, 223
Female Orgasmic Disorder, 32, 135, 136, 138, 139, 141, 142, 195

Female Sexual Arousal Disorder, (FSAD), 31, 71, 104, 116, 117, 123, 194
female sexual dysfunction, 123, 146, 170, 172, 192, 211
fluoxetine, 55, 98, 132, 147
fluvoxamone, 55
Follicle-Stimulating Hormone (FSH), 30
free testosterone, 30
Freud, Sigmund, 3, 7, 18, 19
frigidity, 72, 85
fungal, 82

**G**

gabapentin, 145
generalized type, 32
genetic, 22, 41, 69, 105, 117, 138, 147
genitals, 11, 36, 70, 138, 140, 141, 180, 208
genital pain, 82, 149, 150, 151, 162, 168, 196
genograms, 24
GHB, 61
Goldstein, Irwin, vii, 4
Grafenberg spot (G-spot), 38, 139, 146
group psychotherapy, 37

**H**

heart disease, 23, 64, 72, 77, 120, 137, 197, 204
herbal, 93, 133, 174, 175, 177, 179
herbal treatments, 133
herpes, 83, 186, 220
HIV, 69, 90, 221, 222
homeopathy, 173, 174, 187, 188
homosexuality, 218, 219, 220
hormonal profile, 202
hormone replacement therapy, 119, 205, 212

hymen, 153
hyperactive sexual desire, 97, 99
hyperprolactinemia, 69, 71, 81
hypertension, 23, 49
hypnotherapy, 159
Hypoactive Sexual Desire Disorder, 31, 68, 88, 89, 98, 194
hypogonadism, 23
hypothalamus, 1, 45, 47, 178, 179
hysterectomy, 70, 72, 169, 206

**I**

Ignarro, Louis, Ph.D., vii, xi, xv, xvi, 2, 4, 43
illicit drugs, 28, 49, 97, 106, 117
implants, 33, 35, 79
impotence, 52, 53, 58, 61, 78, 86, 131, 183, 197, 208
incest, 90, 95
individual psychotherapy, 37, 121, 134, 165
injections, 33, 40, 78, 84, 109, 113, 114
injuries, 57, 69, 80, 106, 129, 137, 198, 213
InterStim®, 140
interview, 91, 95, 155
introitus, 152, 160

**K**

Kaplan, Helen Singer, 8, 87, 193
Kegel exercises, 84, 156, 164
Kinsey, Alfred, 3, 215, 218
Kinsey Report, 215

**L**

L-arginine, 74
labial engorgement, 194
laboratory, 30, 50, 57, 67, 68, 71, 73, 91, 95, 126, 131, 213, 220

lactation, 152
Leiblum, Sandra, 7, 8, 15, 19, 70, 85,
    97, 100, 101, 122, 156, 158, 159,
    160, 162, 163, 166, 169
leptin, 130
Levitra (*see vardenafil*)
libido, 8, 9, 17, 48, 52, 54, 58, 59, 61,
    71, 76, 90, 106, 112, 154, 182,
    183, 193, 198, 202, 204, 205
lifelong, 32, 89, 94, 105, 117, 127, 136,
    143, 148, 151, 160
lifetime, vii, 27, 218, 219
limbic system, 1
lordosis, 44, 45, 46
lovemaking, 175, 176, 181, 184, 185
lubricants, 84, 156
lubricating, 94, 160
lubrication-swelling response, 103,
    104, 116, 117, 118
Luteinizing Hormone (LH), 30

## M

Male Erectile Disorder, 31, 35, 68, 73,
    103, 104, 105, 117
Male Orgasmic Disorder, 32, 81, 125,
    126, 142, 143, 145
marijuana, 58, 59
massage, 175, 181
mastectomy, 70, 72
Masters (William) and Johnson
    (Virginia), 1, 3, 8, 10, 14, 15, 18,
    35, 36, 38, 115, 129, 134, 141,
    144, 216
masturbation, 45, 60, 63, 81, 92, 97,
    138, 141, 156, 195, 217, 226, 227
MDMA (ecstasy), 60
meditation, 173, 175
menopause, 23, 28, 73, 92, 118, 137,
    194, 197, 198, 206, 207
Meyer, Adolf, 21
mirtazapine, 55, 56, 93
moclobemide, 55

molestation, 90, 95
monoamine oxidase inhibitors, 49
multiple orgasms, 135, 160
musculature, 45, 47, 150, 160
MUSE®, 35
myocardial infarction, 72, 77, 85

## N

National Health and Social Life
    Survey, 3, 89, 94, 136, 142, 192,
    217
nefazodone, 55
Neoplastic, 69
neoplastic, 69
neurological, 23, 28, 29, 30, 69
neuromodulation, 122, 140
Neurontin, 145
nicotine, 57, 61, 62
nitric oxide, xv, 1, 46
nitroglycerin, 208
noradrenergic, 75, 130, 139
norepinephrine, 44

## O

obesity, 75
Olanzapine, 57
opioids, 61
oral stimulation, 160
orgasm, 8, 9, 12, 13, 18, 27, 45, 50, 65,
    126, 147, 148, 178, 213
orgasmic cephalgia, 126, 145
Oriental medicine, 173, 175
outcome, 39, 41
oxytocin, 1, 46, 63, 64, 139, 144, 147

## P

painful coitus, 151
painful sex, 82, 83, 150
panic disorder, 95, 96
Papavarine, 35

parasympathetic, 14, 107, 108, 109, 207
paroxetine, 55, 131, 132, 148
PDE-5, 2, 33
pellets, 33, 40, 79, 113, 204
pelvic blood flow, 197
penile prosthesis, 114, 115
performance anxiety, 129, 200
Periactin, 56
persistent, 88, 94, 105, 117, 125, 126, 127, 136, 143
peyronie's disease, 23
pH, 30, 72, 196
pharmacological, 2, 4, 41, 64, 116, 121, 122, 146, 212
phentolamine, 35, 207
pheromones, 184
phobia, 99, 130, 147, 161, 162
Phosphodiestrase–5 inhibitors, 33
physical intimacy, 158
pituitary, 23, 46, 69, 71, 106, 178, 198
plateau, 8, 9, 11, 17
poppers, 61
post-menopausal, 17
post-traumatic stress disorder, 96
pregnancy, 24, 28, 49, 58, 73, 83, 129, 152, 153
premature ejaculation, 32, 81, 125, 126, 127, 145, 186
priapism, 59, 60, 65, 106, 114
progesterone, 48
Progestins, 48
Prolactin, 30, 45
Prostaglandins, 47
Prostaglandin E1, 30, 207
prostate, 13, 29, 48, 79, 80, 81, 108, 109, 130, 133, 145, 183
prostate-specific antigen (PSA), 109
prostatectomy, 79, 80, 81
Prostatitis, 130
psychiatric disorders, 22, 23, 130
psychosexual, 154
psychosexual, 154, 170, 210
pubococcygeus, 140, 160, 198

**Q**

Quetiapine, 57

**R**

rape, 61, 90, 95, 161
rapid ejaculation, 126, 148
rectum, 29, 61, 83, 195
resolution, 8, 9, 13, 18
retrograde ejaculation, 126, 143, 145
rigidity, 30, 53, 73, 104, 109, 158

**S**

Sadock, Virginia, vii, 26, 49, 71, 81, 82, 84, 97
selective serotonin reuptake inhibitors, 49, 65, 82, 148
self-help groups, 97, 98
self-stimulation, 135, 156
Sensate focus, 35, 36
serotonin, 2, 44
sertraline, 55, 132
sex,
    education, 40, 159
    hormone-binding globulin, 30
    hormones, 47
    steroids, 89, 90
    surrogates, 38, 41
    therapy, 35, 144
sexual,
    dissatisfaction, 200
    health, xv, xvi, 2, 4, 100, 141, 142, 146, 192, 210, 213
    interaction, 7, 9, 15, 158
    medicine, iv, 1, 3, 5, 142
    positions, 38, 131
    response cycle, 2, 3, 7, 8, 14, 15, 18, 54, 87, 193, 201
    satisfaction, 9, 15, 16, 53, 138, 147, 199
    tension, 9, 10, 12
    trauma, 95, 121, 153, 161, 200, 202

Sexual Arousal Disorders, xi, 8, 31, 35, 103, 104, 195
Sexual Aversion Disorder, 31, 88, 93, 94, 98, 194
Sexual Desire Disorders, 31
Sexual Dysfunction Due to a General Medical Condition, 31
sildenafil, 2, 33, 78, 92, 112, 122
situational, 27, 32, 82, 87, 105, 116, 136, 138, 142, 158, 194, 195, 200, 201, 210
smoking, 23, 49, 61, 77, 106, 129, 193, 197
spasm, 12, 150, 154, 155, 160, 171, 197
squeeze method, 131
SSRI-induced sexual dysfunction, 32, 55, 56, 139, 144
SSRIs, 54, 55, 56, 93, 98, 104, 121, 132, 133, 137, 139, 200, 203
start and stop method, 134
substance, xi, 22, 23, 25, 28, 31, 32, 40, 43, 50, 62, 106, 117, 118
Substance-Induced Sexual Dysfunction, 28, 31, 43, 50
sympathetic, 108
systematic desensitization, 141, 164

**T**

tadalafil, 2, 46, 54, 110, 111, 112, 123, 133
Tantric Buddhism, 175
testosterone, 30, 47, 92, 120, 204, 205
Thioridazine, 143, 145
topical anesthetic agents, 132
topical testosterone, 205
total testosterone, 30
traumatic, 69
tumescence, 30, 73, 104, 110
twins, 22

**U**

ultrasound, 157

**V**

vacuum devices, 78, 81
vaginal,
    dilatation, 84, 164
    lubrication, 11
vaginismus, 32, 83, 86, 149, 150, 151, 160, 161, 164, 167, 168, 169, 172, 197
vardenafil, 2, 46, 54, 110, 111, 123, 133
vasocongestion, 10, 11, 16, 103, 116, 118, 199
venlafaxine, 55
Viagra, (see sildenafil)
viral, 82
visual analogue, 156
vomeronasal organ, 184
vulva, 36, 152, 196
vulvodynia, 157, 168, 172, 195, 212, 213

**W**

warts, 83
Wellbutrin, 56, 92
worry, 95, 100, 226, 227

**Y**

yohimbine, 44, 56, 207

**Z**

ziprasidone, 57

Printed in the United States
122753LV00003B/133-138/A